KETO VEGAN

The Complete Guide to Plant-Based Ketogenic Diet: all the secrets to lose weight and increase energy by purifying your body

CONTENTS

INTRODUCTION

The ketogenic diet is just a high fat diet that generally seems to benefit a few individuals who have epilepsy, particularly kids. It's perhaps not just a magical cure but 1 solution to this assorted anti-epileptic medications available. Even the ketogenic diet delivers the benefit of improved seizure control for a number of kids, and sometimes, improved mental alertness with fewer medications. The ketogenic diet is frequently considered a tricky regimen to follow along, but together with exercise, and also an understanding exactly what the dietary plan intends to reach, it might be reduced into a regular pattern. The simple intention is to modify your system's primary fuel source of carbs (such as sugar and bread) to fats. That is carried out by increasing the consumption of carbs and greatly reducing the consumption of carbs. The actual issue is the diet isn't so restrictive, so which foods eaten should really be considered out to some few a gram throughout meal prep, and a participant might well not eat anything that's not "prescribed "by the dietician. The degree of carbs enabled is low so that the little quantity of sugar in the majority of liquid or chewable medications will protect against the daily diet out of working. As examples, a normal meal could incorporate some sort of meat using vegetables cooked using a carrot sauce plus lots of butter. Heavy lotion might be contained on the medial side for drinking. Still another meal could contain eggs and bacon with a great deal of oil or butter included, and thick cream to beverage. A rather large proportion of carbohydrates must be kept using a low overall calories to that diet to become prosperous.

But isn't fat bad for you personally? Fats are the main topic of a whole lot of terrible press in the past couple of decades. Additionally lots of "healthy "foods have been promoted with a non-fat content...after all "cholesterol kills "does it not? The fact will be much more technical. It's correct that an excessive amount of fat may result in arteriosclerosis (blockages of the arteries), that may result in heart attacks or strokes, however fats even provide an important function to perform in nutrient health. Cholesterol in controlled levels is important and also maybe not as awful as humans are educated. The function of their dietary importance is shared fully to know that the ketogenic diet program. To now, be assured, the high fat content of the ketogenic diet have not yet been demonstrated to be detrimental.

CHAPTER ONE

WHAT'S THE KETO DIET?

The keto diet involves going long bouts on exceptionally low (no more than 30g every day) to nearly zero gram each day of carbohydrates and upping your own carbs to really a large degree (to the stage at which they can constitute just as much as 65 percent of one's everyday macro-nutrients in take.) The concept behind that would be to get the body to a state of ketosis. Within this condition of ketosis that the human body is assumed to become more prone to make use of fat to energy- and - research states that it will not only this. Depleting your own carbohydrate/glycogen liver stores and moving fat for fuel means you should wind up being shredded.

Then you follow this simple stage from say Monday before sat 12pm (day) (or sat 7pm, depending on which version you see). Then using that time before 12 midnight Sunday night (up to 3-6 hours after) do your huge carbohydrate up...

(a few state, and this is also ordered from your physique, you can go nuts at the carbohydrate up and eat whatever you need and there are people who wisely- in my opinion - recipe nevertheless adhering into the sterile carbohydrates even throughout your carbohydrate.)

Therefore calculating your amounts is as easy as the next...

Calculate your required maintenance amount of daily calories...

(if you're looking to shed quickly use 1-3 - that wouldn't advise this, even if you'd like an even far more flat drop in your body fat usage 1-5 of course in the event that you will really try to sustain or put on a muscle mass subsequently utilize 17)

Human body fat in pounds x15 = a

Protein to your own afternoon 1g per weight in pounds= b

Bx4=c (c) amount of calories allocated to a everyday protein allowance).

A c = id (id = level of carbs to be allocated to fat ingestion).

D/9= gram every day of fat to become swallowed.

The ending calculation should render you having a quite large number for the own fat intake.

Now for all those of you wondering energy levels... Notably for training because you can find not any carbohydrates, together with there being such a higher quantity of fat from the diet you truly feel quite saturated along with the fat can be just a really great fuel source for the human system. (One variant I have made will be to already have a wonderful fish noodle roughly one hour or so until I train and that I believe it is gives me enough energy to make it through my work) (I'm mindful of the arguments designed to have fats 2 3 hrs differently of training. While I won't have carbs 2 3 hrs after training like I desire quick absorption and blood flow afterward I find no problem with slowing down everything until training therefore that my own body gets use of a slow-digesting energy-source).

Continuing with general principles...

You will find several that state to get a 30g carbohydrate intake instantly after training- only enough to fulfill liver glycogen levels. And there are the ones which state having much as this can push you out of ketosis- that the condition you're working to keep up. Because I have completed the post workout shake for that past 8years of my practice that I have opted to try out the "no post workout "course! I guess that I might also try!

Within my carbohydrate upward period- to the interest of the who'd love to learn about you're able to get fit and sill eat exactly the things you would like (in moderation)- to first fourteen days I am relaxed by what I eat within this era however the subsequent 6 weeks I shall just eat carbs that are clean.

A concise summary of this ketogenic diet

The ketogenic diet, colloquially referred to as the keto diet is a favorite diet containing high levels of carbs, sufficient protein and very low carbohydrate. It's likewise known as a low carb-high fat (lchf) diet and a very low carbohydrate diet plan.

It had been mostly formulated for the treatment of epilepsy which didn't answer medications to the disorder.

The diet has been originally released in 1921 by dr. Russell wilder at the mayo clinic. Dr. Wilder found that placing psychiatric patients onto an easy failed to decrease the frequency of these indicators. During its book, there weren't many different alternatives out there for the cure of epilepsy.

The ketogenic diet was broadly used for its upcoming two years in treating epilepsy both in kids and adults. In a number of epilepsy studies, roughly 50 percent of patients reported with at least 50% decrease in seizures.

Nevertheless, that the advent of anticonvulsant medication in the 1940s and then introduced the ketogenic diet into an "alternative "medicine. Most healthcare givers in addition to patients, also found it a good deal simpler to make use of the pills when compared with adhering to the strict ketogenic diet plan. It had been then ignored from the cure of epilepsy by the majority of pros.

Back in 1993, a revived interest from the ketogenic diet has been triggered by Hollywood producer Jim Abrahams. Abraham had his two yrs of age boy, Charlie, attracted into the johns Hopkins hospital to get epilepsy therapy. Charlie undergone rapid transplant control over days of working with the ketogenic diet plan.

Jim Abrahams established the Charlie foundation in 1994 that helped revive research campaigns. His production of this television picture named "first do no harm "starring Meryl Streep additionally helped greatly boost the ketogenic diet plan.

The foods were built to present the human body with the ideal amount of nourishment it needs for repair and growth. The calculation of the sum of consumed calories has been achieved to give sufficient quantities that'll soon be in a position to encourage and keep the appropriate burden essential for that child's weight and height reduction.

Underlying concepts of this ketogenic diet

The timeless ketogenic diet features a "fat " to a "mix of carbohydrates and protein " percentage of 4:1.

The overall daily caloric break down of this ketogenic diet plan is the following:

60-80percent of calorie consumption

2025 percent from proteins

510 percent from carbohydrates

The proportion of this foods at a ketogenic diet plan is formulated to help your system cause and sustain a condition of ketosis.

Nevertheless, that the ketogenic landscape has enlarged significantly both in its implementation and application. As the classical ketogenic diet remains widely used now, it's formed the foundation for its evolution of several other ketogenic protocols.

Ketogenic diet plans ostensibly encourage the ingestion of roughly 20 to 50 g of carbs every day. Protein ingestion is mild and mostly is dependent upon factors like the sex, height, activity levels of the person. Essentially, the total calorie of this diet plan is balanced chiefly predicated on the sum of fat.

The fat and also protein ratios at a ketogenic diet

Enriched healthy fat intake is the most important focus of this ketogenic dietplan. Additionally, the objective is to keep up their condition of ketosis in any way times hence enabling the human body to make use of greater excess fat.

Your system digests protein and fat otherwise. Fat is possibly your human body's most useful supply of energy and also at a condition of ketosis, your human body is able to take advantage of body fat and dietary fat evenly well.

Generally, fats have very small effect on glucose and insulin production in the human own body. But, protein affects both these levels if consumed in huge amounts beyond what the human system requires.

Approximately 56 percent of those excess ingested protein is converted into sugarlevels. It's the result of upsetting that the ketosis condition of much burning like a consequence of your human body responding to the sugar generated by the protein breakdown.

Based upon your own type and origin of ingested fats, a highfat diet might be a lot fitter. Reducing carbohydrate intake and increasing your usage of saturated fats out of mostly medium-chain Efas may really enhance the own body's profile.

The ketogenic diet raises hdl (good) cholesterol levels while at the exact same time reduces cholesterol levels. Both of these facets are the chief markers for cardiovascular illness.

A ratio of compared to 2.0 on your triglyceride-to-hdl ratio usually means that you're succeeding. Nevertheless, the closer this ratio is to 1.0 or lower, the fitter your heart.

This type of fat profile is connected with greater security against heart attacks and other cardiovascular issues.

Consumption of increased lean protein at the lack of sufficient levels of carbs in the diet could cause "bunny starvation "rabbit starvation can be just a state where there's an insufficient number of fats. This illness has been observed in food diets which mostly contain fats.

One of those important indicators of bunny starvation is nausea. The nausea may usually come to be serious and might result in departure. This frequently occurs over the initial 3 days to a week of pure lean diets. If sufficient quantities of fats aren't absorbed at the achievement days, the nausea may worsen and could result in dehydration and potential departure.

Keto diet and some breakdowns?

The keto diet, also abbreviated by ketogenic, is really a especially lowcarb, highfat diet that is very like additional lowcarb food diets, including the Atkins approach. Even the keto diet drastically reduces caloric consumption when substituting your human body's most important energy sources. This decline in carbohydrate usage leads your system to some metabolic condition called ketosis.

If this happens, your metabolic rate starts to burn up fat. This course of action is indeed unbelievably effective, it can help weight loss alongside other health and fitness benefits. The not-so-obvious benefits of eating keto foods are increasingly being famished less frequently and using a steady sum of energy. This will definitely help you to stay sharp and focused throughout your afternoon.

Ketogenic diet plans are characterized with a huge decline in blood sugar levels and insulin levels. Sugar may be your mind's key food, but the brain may be fed up together with ketones, which can be made out of fat from the liver.

For many people, ingestion keto diet appears to be somewhat safe. But, it's still contentious and also three kinds of individuals need special concern: patients with diabetes who take medications including insulin, individuals who have higher blood pressure onto anti-hypertensive medications, and breast feeding women. In such scenarios, it's excellent to find a physician and rate your wellness insurance and adapt medications before beginning the keto dietplan.

Different types of ketogenic diet plans

You will find several variations of this ketogenic diet regime, for example:

- Standard ketogenic diet (skd): this really is an incredibly lowcarb, moderate-protein and highfat dietplan. It generally comprises 75 percent fat, 20 percent protein and just 5 percent carbohydrates.

- Cyclical ketogenic diet (ckd): this diet calls for periods of higher-carb re-feeds, for example as for instance 5 ketogenic days accompanied by two highcarb days.

- Targeted ketogenic diet (tkd): this diet lets you incorporate carbohydrates around workouts.

- Highprotein ketogenic diet this is somewhat like a typical ketogenic dietplan, however, comprises greater protein. The ratio is frequently 60 percent fat, 35 percent protein and 5 percent carbohydrates.

But, just the conventional and noninvasive ketogenic diet plans are studied broadly. Cyclical or concentrated ketogenic diet plans are somewhat more advanced level approaches and chiefly used by athletes or bodybuilders.

So what would you consume about a keto diet?

Listed below are the keto foods you can eat on this dietplan, sprinkled by carbohydrate content per 100 g (in ascending order):

- Natural fats such as butter and coconut oil (0 gram of carbohydrates)

- Meat (0 grams of carbohydrates)

- Fish and fish (0 gram of carbohydrates)

- Eggs (1) gram of carbohydrates)

- Cheese along with other dairy products (1) gram of carbohydrates)

- Veggies which grow over earth (1 5 gram of carbohydrates)

What should you avoid to a keto diet?

And below would be the foods which keep you from achieving ketosis, sprinkled by carbohydrate content per 100 g (in descending order):

- Candy (70 gram of carbohydrates)

- Chocolate pubs (60 gram of carbohydrates)

- Donuts (49 gram of carbohydrates)

- Bread (4 6 gram of carbohydrates)

- Pasta (2-9 gram of carbohydrates)

- Rice (28 gram of carbohydrates)

- Soda/juice (10 gram of carbohydrates)

- Fresh fruit (6-20 gram of carbohydrates)

- Veggies which grow below floor (7-17 gram of carbohydrates)

- Beer (4 gram of carbohydrates)

Advantages of a keto diet meal plan

A keto diet provides many health benefits like those of additional lowcarb food diets, however, it generally seems to optimize these benefits:

- Weight reduction

- Reduced body weight percent

- Calmer gut

- Control within the appetite

- Charge of bloodstream sugar and also the prospect of reversing type two diabetes

- Increased energy and psychological performance

- Improved wellbeing markers (hdl, triglycerides)

- Enriched physical endurance

Several studies have shown that keto meals may provide benefits for different health issues, specially such as metabolic, neurological, or even insulin-related diseases. What's more, the ketogenic diet was created to take care of neurological disorders like epilepsy.

A number of those diseases which may be influenced favorably by changing to keto are recorded below:

Heart disorder -- by decreasing risk factors like bodyfat, hdl cholesterol levels, higher blood pressure, and high blood sugar.

Cancer by slowing the tumor development.

Alzheimer's disorder -- by lessening the signs and slowing the development.

Epilepsy -- by reducing the amount of seizures in children.

Parkinson's disorder -- by accentuating the signs.

Polycystic ovary infection -- by lowering insulin amounts.

Brain accidents -- by helping recovery following a brain injury or concussion (just creature studies).

Acne -- by lowering insulin amounts and thanks to eating less sugar and processed food items.

Steps to begin the keto diet

You will find several natural maxims you ought to follow:

- Expel carbohydrates from your daily diet plan.

- Limit protein ingestion -- keep in mind this is a lowcarb diet program however, maybe not just a high-protein.

- Utilize fat to assist you reach ketosis.

- Drink a lot of water to prevent dehydration.

- Maintain electrolytes, notably salt.

- Eat just when you're hungry.

- Educate your meals based on keto recipes.

- Focus on entire foods rather than processed ones.

- Exercise regularly.

A keto diet may be simple if you learn a few basic abilities, like how to organize easy and fun meals, the way to incorporate more carbohydrates in your daily diet plan, and also just how to eat and stay keto.

The way to find yourself in ketosis

The main objective of all that the keto diet will be always to get to ketosis, i.e.and allow the own body to begin burning off fat. How would you do so? To begin with, the absolute most crucial issue is always to restrict carbs to 20 grams every day or not. This condition fulfills the strict lowcarb keto dietary basics. But, soluble fiber (that's a carbohydrate) must not be limited as it helps in achieving ketosis. If you're not certain just how much 20 g of carbohydrates is also, you may utilize published keto diet programs and meal plans that are designed with over 20 g of carbohydrates. Ergo, no counting is demanded.

The fantastic news is that simply restricting carbohydrates to create some amount of lack finally leads to ketosis. To be satisfied with your keto diet outcomes, you must experience some extra steps, such as controlling your daily caloric intake and increasing your fat intake.

Secondly, your protein consumption ought to be restricted by moderate levels as excess protein is converted into sugar in your system, diminishing ketosis. Accordingly, approximately 1.5 g of protein per kilogram of bodyweight each day are enough in the event that you would like to keep a suitable dietplan.

Third eating enough fat is essential to staying fulfilled. In the event that you add irregular fasting, ketosis should come faster faster, however unlike appetite, then a keto diet plan is sustainable and also may cause you to feel great. 1 option if you're feeling hungry all of the time will be always to add extra fat (olive, coconut oil, etc.) On meals.

How long can it have to become involved with ketosis?

Should you stay below your typical amount of caloric ingestion, then you definitely should attain a condition of ketosis in just three or two, though in a few instances upto seven. The fastest solution to get involved with ketosis will be always to exercise and fast, which arouses the ingestion of nourishment on the human entire body. This will enhance your glucose reservations and change your metabolic process towards burning off fat.

A keto diet program for beginners could be initiated by eating excess fat to speed upbringing on the ketosis condition. Simultaneously, you need to start reducing processed carbohydrates. Still another option, however a hard one to do, would be always to drink just water for a couple days.

Excreting ketones in urine can be a sure sign you are in ketosis. But to see whether you are init special ketosis strips which determine if ketones come from the urine may be properly used. A little an invasive and expensive strategy is to start looking for ketones in your blood having a blood ketone meter.

What're the indicators to be in ketosis?

Many folks who begin a ketogenic diet may feel some disagreeable symptoms, referred to as "keto influenza " these signs begin several days once you begin the daily diet plan, plus they comprise, but are not limited to, these:

- Light nausea

- Headache

- Infection

- Dizziness

- Difficulty focusing ("brain fog ")

- Deficiency of motivation

- Irritability

But these first ketosis symptoms disappear as the body adjusts to enhanced fat burning off. Usually, the version takes approximately weekly.

The motives these flu-like symptoms occur are connected to greater water excretion, ordinary after formerly keeping water out of absorbing carb-rich food items. You can even notice increased bleeding and also a lack in extra salt, too. This causes dehydration and also a deficiency of salt. These procedures might also be behind many influenza symptoms.

But these indications of ketosis might be relieved or prevented from drinking enough water and drinking salt. An easy remedy to those flu-like outward symptoms would be to drink bouillon or broth at least one time every day.

Other common keto diet sideeffects

You will find additional more common negative effects, the majority that is looked at a normally negative encounter. But, getting more salt and water can be useful for these unwanted side effects too.

Other facet effects comprise:

- Keto breath which smells like nail polish remover (acetone can be really a ketone)

- Metallic taste in the mouth

- Leg cramps

- Constipation

- Heart palpitations

- Paid off tolerance to alcohol

- Appetite suppression

- Scrub hair loss

- Elevated cholesterol

- Keto rash

- Greater flaxseed blood sugar

- Gout

- Gall-stone issues

Strategies for maintaining a keto meal-plan

- Jump foods -- considering breakfast because the main meal of your afternoon might be readily shifted when with this diet program. If you are not blasting whenever you awaken, then you can skip breakfast, then catch a fast keto shake, or even have a walk. A lowered desire is a frequent quality of the daily diet plan, therefore skipping dinner isn't a issue. But in the event that you're hungry once you wake up but are brief time, then a keto breakfast can be yummy, satisfying, and easy to get ready.

- Educate your personal meals -- delicious meals for dinner or lunch is readily prepared by adding fish or meat with a salad, such as. A vegetarian keto diet can be an option--e.g. Vegetables cooked using melted cheese, butter, or perhaps a rich sauce.

- Stock upon keto veggies -- all these include spinach, celery, asparagus, avocado, zucchini, cauliflower, cabbage, pineapple, broccoli, spinach, Brussels sprouts. Because you can see, the majority of these are still green! Plus so they grow above earth. That really is quick method to inform that vegetable contains too many carbohydrates.

- Replace bread -- unsurprisingly, bread is among the very familiar foods that people overlook with this particular diet regime. But fear not there are a number of yummy recipes to get keto bread that will be low in carbohydrates to become acceptable with this particular diet program.

- Dine-out -- if you are dining outside, avoid foods such as pasta or bread and also ask foods with excess fat (i.e., olive or coconut oil) should you require it.

- Eat clever -- choose food that is real rather than specifically "low-fat " services and products. Your purpose needs to be to stay alive, not merely shed weight.

- Calculate your carbohydrates -- you might also work with a keto calculator to gauge the number of carbohydrates you eat a time, roughly.

- Cannot quit the desserts? -- do not worry, in addition, there are keto desserts. They truly are lower in carbohydrates but still yummy.

- Avoid snacking once you are not hungry -- but eating keto snacks can minimize the damage, plus so they're fine for once you become hungry.

- Heal yourself but proceed to get healthy, moderate-carb choices like berries, berries, seeds and nuts, and chocolates.

- Sleep sufficient -- get a minimum of seven hours each night and continue to keep your stress in check. It has been demonstrated that sleep deprivation and stress hormones increase glucose levels, slowing ketosis and weight reduction, plus so they may possibly make it more difficult to resist temptation and follow your own diet plan.

CHAPTER TWO

HAVE YOU BEEN RIGHT FOR THE KETO DIET?

Nowadays, it may seem like everybody is speaking about the ketogenic (in summary, keto) diet - that the exact low fat, moderate protein diet, highfat diet program which transforms the body into a fat burning machine. Hollywood celebrities and athletes have reported this diet benefits, by reducing weight, lowering blood glucose, fighting inflammation, and reducing cancer risk, rising energy, into slowing aging. What's keto something you need to think about carrying on? These tips will explain exactly what this diet is about, the advantages and disadvantages, in addition to the difficulties to be on the watch for.

Normally, the body uses sugar as the chief supply of gas for electricity. Whenever you're following the keto diet and you're eating not many carbohydrates with just moderate levels of carbs (excess protein might also be altered into carbohydrates), the system exerts its own fuel source to perform mostly on fat. The liver also produces ketones (a form of fatty acid) in the fat) all these ketones turned into an gas supply to the system, notably the brain that absorbs lots of energy and may run using either sugar or ketones.

After the entire body produces ketones, it passes a metabolic condition called ketosis. Fasting may be the simplest means to attain ketosis. Whenever you're eating or fasting not many carbohydrates and just moderate levels of protein, the body turns to burning off stored fat. That's the reason why folks have a tendency to lose excess weight to the keto dietplan.

The keto diet plan is perhaps not brand new. It was found from the 1920s as a clinical therapy to treat epilepsy in children, however if anti-epileptic medication came into the current market, the dietary plan dropped into obscurity until recently. Considering its success in lessening the quantity of seizures in elderly patients, a growing number of research is done on the capability of the daily diet to deal with a range of psychiatric ailments and other kinds of chronic disorders.

Neuro-degenerative diseases. New research suggests that the great things about keto from Alzheimer's, Parkinson's, dementia, as well as multiple sclerosis (ms). It might also be protective from traumatic brain injury and stroke. 1 notion for keto's neuroprotective effects is the ketones produced throughout ketosis provide additional fuel into cells, which might help those cells withstand the damage from inflammation due to these diseases.

Fat and weight reduction. If you're trying to drop weight, that the keto diet is very effective since it will help to gain access and discard the own body fat. Constant appetite may be the largest difficulty when you attempt to shed weight. Even the keto diet will help to avoid this problem as reducing carbohydrate intake and increasing fat ingestion promote satiety, which makes it a lot easier for visitors to abide by diet. In a report, obese test subjects shed twice the quantity of fat in 2 4 weeks moving to a lowcarb diet (20.7 pounds) in comparison to this group on a low-carb diet (10.5 pounds).

Type two diabetes. Apart from weight reduction, the keto diet also will help enhance insulin sensitivity, which is perfect for anybody with type two diabetes. In a study published in nutrition & metabolism, researchers noticed that girls that ate low-fat keto diet plans had the ability to greatly lessen their reliance upon diabetes drugs and can reverse it. In addition, it enhances other wellness markers such as lowering triglyceride levels and ldl (bad) cholesterol and increasing hdl (good) cholesterol.

Cancer. Many folks are unaware that the cancer cells' key fuel is sugar. This usually means eating the ideal diet might help curb cancer development. Since the keto diet is extremely low in carbohydrates, it found the cancer cells in their own principal supply of gas, that is glucose. After your system produces ketones, the nutritious cells may utilize that as energy however, perhaps not exactly the cancer cells, therefore they're being starved to death. Since 1987, studies on keto food diets also have already shown decreased tumor development and improved survival for any range of cancers.

Assessing traditional American, American, paleo, & keto food diets

The main distinction between the keto diet and also the normal American or paleo diet plans is that it contains much fewer carbohydrates and a whole lot more fat. The keto diet ends in ketosis with circulating ketones which range from 0.5-5.0 m m. This could be quantified with a home blood ketone track with ketone test strips. (please be aware that analyzing ketones in urine isn't true)

The way to formulate a keto diet

Inch. Carbs

For many people, to attain ketosis (becoming ketones above 0.5 millimeters) takes one to restrict carbohydrates to somewhere within 2050 g (g)daily. The true number of carbohydrates will differ from one individual to another. In general, the more insulin-resistant a man or woman is, the more resistant they are to ketosis. Some insulin sensitive athletes working aggressively could eat up over 50 g/day and stay in ketosis, where as individuals who have type 2 diabetes and insulin resistance might want to be more closer to 20 30 g/day.

When calculating carbohydrates, one is permitted to make use of carbs, meaning total carbohydrates minus fiber and sugar alcohols. The idea of net carbohydrates is to comprise only carbohydrates that increase blood glucose and insulin. Fiber doesn't need any hormonal or metabolic impact therefore do many sugar alcohols. The exclusion is maltitol that may possess a non-trivial effect on blood sugar levels and insulin. Ergo, if maltitol is really on the part list, then sugar should not be deducted from carbohydrates.

The degree of carbohydrates you may eat up and stay in ketosis can also change with time based upon keto adaptation, weight reduction, exercise habits, medications, etc.. For that reason, an individual ought to quantify their ketone degrees on a regular basis.

Concerning this in general dietplan, carb-dense foods such as pastas, cereals, potatoes, legumes, carbonated candy, carbonated drinks, sodas, and beer aren't suitable.

Most milk products contain carbohydrates in the shape of lactose (milk sugar). But some have less carbohydrates and will be employed regularly. These generally include hard cheeses (parmesan, cheddar), tender, high-grade cheeses (brie), full-fat cream cheese, heavy whipping cream, and sour cream.)

A carbohydrate level less than 50 g/day generally reduces to these:

5 10 g carbohydrates out of protein-based food items. Eggs, cheese, and shell fish will hold a couple residual g of carbohydrates from sources and also added marinades and spices.

1015 g carbohydrates from non-starchy veggies.

5 10 g carbohydrates out of nuts/seeds. Most nuts feature 5 6 gram carbohydrates per oz.

5 10 g carbohydrates from fruits such as tomatoes, cauliflower, tomatoes, and avocados.

5 10 g carbohydrates from mixed sources like low-fat desserts, highfat dressings, or drinks with very tiny levels of sugar.

Beverages

Most folks require at the least half of a gallon of overall fluid every day. The very best sources include filtered water, organic tea and coffee (regular and decaf, unsweetened), also un-sweetened coconut and almond milk. Diet carbonated drinks and drinks are best avoided since they contain artificial sweeteners. In case you drink white or red wine, then limit to 1 2 glasses, then the drier the better. Should you drink spirits, then steer clear of the refrigerated mixed beverages.

2. Protein

A keto diet plan is not a higher protein diet. The main reason is that protein increases insulin and will be converted into sugar by means of a process known as gluconeogenesis, thus, inhibiting ketosis. But a keto diet shouldn't be excessively low in protein as it often leads to lack in muscular tissues and function.

The typical adult requires approximately 0.8-1.5 gram per kilogram (kilogram) of lean body mass each day. It's crucial to generate the calculation based on lean body mass, not body weight reduction. The main reason is basically because fat does not demand protein to keep up, just the muscle mass.

By way of example, should an person weighs 150 pounds (roughly 150/2.2 = 68.18 kg) and features a body fat content of 20 percent (or lean body mass of 80 percent = 68.18 kg x 0.8 = 54.55 kg), the protein demand might vary between 44 (= 54.55 x 0.8) into 82 (= 54.55 x 1.5) g/day.

People that are insulin immune or doing exactly the keto diet for curative reasons (cancer, epilepsy, etc.) Should target to be nearer to the decrease protein limitation. The higher limitation is for all those that are very athletic or active. For all who is utilizing the keto diet for fat reduction or other health and fitness benefits, the sum of daily protein is somewhere between.

Most useful resources of premium excellent protein incorporate:

Organic, pastured eggs (6 8 gram of protein/egg)

Grass fed meats (6 9 gram of protein/oz)

Animal-based sources of omega3 fats, for example as for instance wild-caught such as mackerel, mackerel, and anchovies, and herrings. (6 9 gram of protein/oz)

Seeds and vegetables, such as macadamia, almonds, pecans, flaxseeds, and sesame seeds. (4 8 gram of protein/quarter cup)

Veggies (1 2 gram of protein/oz)

3. Fat

Having guessed out the precise levels of protein and carbs to consume, and the remaining part of the diet stems from fat. A keto diet plan is high in fat. When adequate fat is eaten and bodyweight is maintained. If weight-loss is desired, an individual needs to consume less fat and then count on stored bodyfat for energy expenditure alternatively.

For people who eat 2000 calories each day to keep their weight, daily fat intakes are approximately 156-178 g/day. For very busy people who have higher energy conditions that are maintaining fat intakes may possibly even transcend 300 g/day.

Many folks can withstand high intakes of fat, however certain states like gall bladder removal might influence the total amount of fat which could be consumed at one meal. In this instance, more frequent meals or usage of bile salts or gastrointestinal enzymes saturated in lipase could be useful.

Avoid eating undesirable fats like trans fat, exceptionally processed polyunsaturated vegetable oils, in addition to elevated levels of omega6 poly unsaturated fats.

Best meals to obtain premium quality fats involve:

- Avocados and coconut oil

- Coconuts and coconut oil

- Grass fed butter, ghee, and steak fat

- Organic, pastured thick lotion

- Jojoba oil

- Lard out of pastured pigs

- Moderate chain triglycerides (MCTS)

MCT is really a specific kind of fat that's metabolized differently in routine fatty acids that are fatty. The liver could utilize MCTS to quickly create energy, before sugar, hence allowing an elevated production of ketones.

Concentrated sources of MCT oil are all available as supplements. Lots of men and women utilize these to help reach ketosis. The single real food that's uniquely full of MCTS is coconut oil. About two thirds of this coconut fat is based from MCT.

Who need to be cautious using a keto diet?

For many people, a keto diet is very safe and sound. But, there are particular people who should take special maintenance and talk with their doctors before you go on this kind of diet plan.

People taking medications such as diabetes. Dosage might have to be corrected as blood sugar levels goes with a lowcarb diet.

People taking medications for hypertension. Dosage might have to be corrected as blood pressure goes with a lowcarb diet.

People that are breastfeeding shouldn't continue an extremely strict lowcarb diet as your body may lose approximately 30 gram of carbohydrates every day via the milk. Consequently, have at least 50 gram of carbohydrates daily whilst still breastfeeding.

People with kidney illness should talk to their doctors before doing a keto dietplan.

Typical concerns using a keto diet

Being able to attain ketosis. Ensure that you aren't eating a lot of protein and there's not any hidden carbohydrates in the packed foods you eat up.

Eating the incorrect forms of fat such as for example the exceptionally elegant polyunsaturated corn and soybean oils.

Indicators of a "keto-flu ", like feeling nervousness, nausea, nausea, fatigue, brain fog, as well as constipation. After in ketosis, your human body has a tendency to excrete more sodium. If a person just isn't getting sufficient sodium out of the daily diet, symptoms of a keto-flu could appear. That is easily remedied by drinking two cups of broth (with additional salt) daily. In case you exercise vigorously and also the perspiration speed is elevated, you might have to incorporate back much more salt.

Dawn effect. Normal fasting blood glucose are somewhat less than 100 mg/dl & a lot of people in ketosis can attain this amount if they're not diabetic. Nevertheless, in certain people fasting blood glucose have a tendency to grow, particularly in the early hours, while to a keto dietplan. That is known as the "dawn effect "and can be brought on to the typical adrenal growth in early cortisol (stress hormone) that stimulates the liver to produce more glucose. If it occurs, make certain you're not consuming excess protein and perhaps not overly near bed time. Stress and inadequate sleep may also contribute to high cortisol levels. If you're insulin resistant, then you can also want additional hours for you to attain ketosis.

Low athletic performance. Keto-adaptation often takes approximately four weeks. Throughout that, rather than accomplishing intense exercise or workouts, switch to a thing that's not as vigorous. After the adaptation period, athletic operation usually contributes to normal and sometimes better still, specially to endurance sports.

Keto-rash is perhaps not a frequent complication of this diet program. Probable causes include production of acetone (an application of ketone) from the perspiration that disturbs skin or nutrient deficiencies including minerals or protein. Shower immediately after exercise and be sure that you eat nutrient dense foods that are whole.

Ketoacidosis. This is a really rare illness which happens when blood ketone levels exceed 1-5 mm. Even a well-formulated keto diet doesn't result in ketoacidosis. Certain conditions like type 1 diabetes, obesity being on medications with sglt-2 inhibitors such as type 2 diabetes, or breast feeding require additional caution. Symptoms include nausea, nausea, vomiting, and rapid shallow breathing. Mild cases might be solved with sodium bicarbonate mixed with orange or apple juice. Acute symptoms need immediate medical care.

Can be keto safe for long-term?

That really is a place of a controversy. Though there have never been some studies suggesting some adverse long-term aftereffects to be to a keto diet, so many experts today think that your human body can create a "immunity " into the advantages of ketosis unless you regularly cycles in and outside of it. Additionally, eating an extremely highfat diet at the longterm might well not be acceptable for many body types.

Cyclical keto diet

As soon as you are able to create over 0.5 mm of ketones in blood onto a frequent basis, it's time to get started digesting carbohydrates back into the diet plan. Rather than eating only 2050 gram of carbs/day, then you might choose to boost it to 100-150 gram on those carb-feeding days. Ordinarily, 2-3 days per week will likely be adequate. Ideally, in addition, this is achieved on intensity training days which you truly increase your daily caloric intake.

This strategy of biking can get the diet regime more suitable for a men and women who're reluctant to permanently eradicate a few of their preferred foods. But, it can also lower fix and devotion to this keto diet or activate binges in vulnerable people.

Is your keto diet right for you?

Are you currently curious in reducing your weight? Are you sick and tired of diets that urge no or low carbohydrates and crave your high fat meats? You could be considering going to the keto diet, the newest kid on the block. Endorsed by lots of celebrities including Halle berry, LeBron James and kimkardashian amongst many others, the keto diet has long become the topic of much disagreement among dietitians and health practitioners. Does one wonder whether the keto diet is safe and best for you personally?

You need to be aware that your system makes use of sugar in the kind of glycogen to work. The keto diet that's incredibly restricted in glucose forces the body to utilize fat as fuel rather than sugar since it doesn't secure sugar levels. After your human body doesn't receive enough sugar to fuel, then the liver is made to show the readily available fat to ketones which can be used by your human body as fuel - ergo the expression ketogenic.

This diet is really a high fat diet with moderate levels of nourishment. Based upon your carbohydrate intake your system reaches a state of ketosis at under weekly and remains there. As fat can be employed rather than glucose to get fuel within the human anatomy, the body weight loss is striking with no presumed restriction of carbs.

The keto diet plan is in a way it you should plan to receive 60-75percent of your daily calorie consumption, 15 30 percent from protein and just 5 10 percent from carbs. This typically means you could eat just 2050 g of carbohydrates a day.

What do you consume on this particular diet plan?

The diet plan is really a high fat diet that's notably like Atkins. But, there are greater focus in fats, usually 'good' fats. To the keto diet you could possess

- Jojoba oil

- Coconut-oil

- Nut oils

- Butter

- Ghee

- Grassfed beef

- Chicken

- Fish

- Other meats

- Full fat milk

- Eggs

- Cream

- Leafy greens

- Non-starchy veggies

- Nuts

- Seeds

You can also get an entire selection of snacks which can be meant for keto followers. Because you can observe in the particular list, veggies are not restricted. You can get low carbohydrate veggies in a limited variety (mainly tomatoes), however might need to forego your favorite veggies since these are typical candy or starchy.

This diet plan comprises no carbohydrates of any sort, starchy veggies such as potatoes (as well as tubers), no sweets or sugar, no cakes and breads, zero legumes and legumes, no pasta, no other pasta and hamburgers and hardly any alcohol. This does mean no coffee with tea or milk with milk - actually, no milk and also ice-creams and milk based desserts.

A lot of them have work-around since you're able to acquire carbohydrate free bread and pizza, so you can possess cauliflower rice now there are restaurants which appeal to keto aficionados.

Which will be the advantages of the keto diet?

In case you're wondering if that nutritional supplement is safe, its own proponents and people who have achieved their weight loss goals will definitely agree it is safe. One of the benefits of the keto diet plan you can anticipate:

- Lack of weight

- Paid off or no. Sugar spikes

- Appetite control

- Seizure restraining effect

- Blood pressure normalizes in elevated blood pressure

- Paid down strikes of migraine

Type2 diabetes patients with this diet could have the ability to lower their medications

A few advantages to people afflicted by cancer

Besides this first four, there's not adequate evidence to back up its efficacy otherwise for different diseases as more research is called for over the longterm.

Are there any some sideeffects with the diet program?

If you initially initiate the keto diet you can suffer with that which is called keto flu. These indicators might not occur in most individuals and usually take up a day or two after being on the diet when the system is at a condition of ketosis. A few of the sideeffects are:

- Nausea

- Cramps and stomach anxiety

- Headache

- Throwing up

- Diarrhoea or constipation

- Muscle cramps

- Dizziness and poor concentrations

- Insomnia

- Carbohydrate and sugar cravings

These can require up to and including week to subside as the body become accustomed to the new diet regimen. It is possible to even have problems with different issues whenever you begin the keto diet - you can realize you have increased bleeding, therefore it's crucial to remain well hydrated. You can also suffer with keto breath as soon as the entire body reaches on optimal ketosis also you're able to work with a mouthwash or brush your teeth frequently.

Usually the unwanted effects are temporary as soon as the human body acclimatizes into the diet, those needs to disappear.

How secure would be that the keto diet?

Exactly like some other dietary plan which limits foods in certain types, the keto diet plan is not without risks. Since you aren't designed to eat lots of vegetables and fruits, lentils and legumes and other foods, as you may suffer with deficiency of several nutrients that are essential. Since this diet is high in fatty foods and, even if you have pleasure into the 'bad' fats, then you can get elevated cholesterol levels increasing your chance of cardiovascular illness.

From the longterm that the keto diet may also cause lots of nutrient deficiencies as you can't eat grains, lots of produce and overlook on fiber as additionally crucial vitamins, minerals, minerals, phytonutrients and antioxidants among other activities. It's possible to suffer with digestive distress, diminished bone density (no milk and also alternative sources of calcium) and liver and kidney issues (the dietary plan places added stress on either organs).

Is your keto diet safe for you personally?

In case you're willing to forego your customary dietary principles and are extremely keen to shed weight, you could well be enticed to check the keto dietplan. The greatest issue of this particular diet plan is poor patient compliance as a result of the carb limitation, and that means you need to make certain you could stay together with the meal choices. In the event that you merely believe it is too tricky to follow along with along with you also can continue a variant of this modified keto diet which gives more carbohydrates.

Nevertheless, that the keto diet plan is unquestionably powerful in assisting you to get rid of weight. As demonstrated by your recent analysis lots of the obese patients followed were successful in reducing your weight. Any issues they faced were also temporary. If you don't need some substantial health issues with the exception of obesity and also have been ineffective in slimming down after any traditional diet, then the keto diet can be a feasible choice. You ought to be entirely determined to drop the weight and also prepare yourself to select a restricted diet specified. Even in the event that you have some health issues, you're able to simply take your physician's advice and also a nutritionist's guidance and proceed with this diet program.

Still another analysis that was performed for a more period demonstrated that moving to the keto diet is beneficial in weight loss and results in lower cholesterol levels using a drop in the cholesterol and an gain in the fantastic cholesterol.

Is your keto diet safe for you personally? Most health practitioners and nutritionists are consented that the keto diet is very good for weight loss loss within the shortterm. In terms of the longterm, more studies are expected. Do remember that obesity isn't a viable choice since it has its risk of medical issues.

Making ketogenic food diets work

The reality

Ketogenic diet plans (more specifically cyclic ketogenic diet plans) would be the best food diets for achieving rapid, ultra-low body fat levels with maximum muscle strength! But just like such general statements that there are real life exceptions. But done correctly - they rarely are the fat loss possible to get a ketogenic diet isn't anything short of astonishing! And, despite what people may tell you personally, you'll even enjoy incredible high energy and general sense of wellness.

The perception

Despite all these promises, more bodybuilders/shapers have experienced negative experiences than ever have experienced favorable outcomes. The primary criticisms are:

- Chronic lethargy

- Unbearable appetite

- Massive de-crease in health operation

- Intense muscle loss

Most these criticisms derive in the failure to heed the caveat previously: ketogenic diet plans have to be carried out correctly! It has to be realised they have been a completely unique metabolic modality that adheres to none of those previously accepted'rules' of fat loss. And there's not any going half way; 50 g of carbohydrates every day and higher protein ingestion isn't ketogenic!

Therefore just how are ketogenic diet plans 'done '? Let's immediately consider how they work out.

Review of ketosis

Just our entire body organs, brain and muscles may utilize either sugar or ketones such as fuel. It's the use of the pancreas and liver (primarily) to modulate that gas provide plus so they reveal a strong prejudice toward adhering with sugar. Glucose may be your 'favorite' fuel since it's derived from prosperity from the diet and also easily obtainable readily from muscle and liver building stores. Ketones need to become deliberately synthesized by the liver but the liver may very quickly synthesize sugar (an activity referred to as 'gluconeogenesis' which uses proteins (protein) or alternative metabolic intermediaries) too.

We do not get beta hydroxybutyrate, acetone, or acetoacetate (ketones) from diet. The liver synthesizes them under duress; as a previous step in terms of acute glucose deprivation such as starvation. For your liver to be surer that ketones would be the arrangement of this afternoon, many requirements must be fulfilled:

- Blood sugar must fall under 50mg/dl

- Low blood sugar must lead to low nourishment and raised glucagon

- Liver glycogen needs to be low or pty'

- A plentiful source of gluconeogenic substrates should not be around

At this stage it is very crucial to say it isn't actually a matter to be'in' or'outside' of ketosis; we do not either completely operate using ketones, or perhaps not. It's a slow and careful glimpse therefore the brain is always and equally dispersed... Ideally. Ketones ought to be stated in tiny levels in blood sugar levels of roughly 60mg/dl. We believe ourselves in ketosis whenever there are greater levels of ketones than sugar in blood.

The truth is that most folks - notably weight coaches - experienced a normal intake of sugar for a fantastic handful of years, at the least. The liver is absolutely effective at producing ketones however, the exceptionally efficient gluconeogenic pathways have the ability to keep low-normal blood sugar over the ketogenic threshold.

Couple this with that the truth that lots of men and women are partially insulin-resistant and have raised fasting insulin (top end of their normal selection (anyhow). Even the bit of blood sugar out of gluconeogenesis induces adequate insulin discharge to dull glucagon output and also the creation of ketones.

Unusual sugar deprivation is going to have the outcome, initially, of overhauling, appetite, fatigue in a lot of people - until ketosis is accomplished. And ketosis won't be reached before liver is made to cease with gluconeogenesis and get started producing ketones. Provided that dietary plan is adequate then a liver will last to generate glucose and perhaps not ketones. This is exactly why no carbohydrate, higher protein diet plans aren't ketogenic.

What's so wonderful around ketosis any way?

Once the body switches up to conducting mostly on ketones lots of very cool things occur:

Lipolysis (body-fat breakdown) is considerably increased

Muscle catabolism (muscle loss) is considerably diminished

Energy amounts are kept in a stable and high condition

Subcutaneous fluid (aka 'water-retention') is expunged

Ostensibly, when we come in ketosis the own body is having fat (ketones) to fuel everything. Therefore, we're not deteriorating muscle to give glucose. In other words, muscle has been researched since it's nothing more to offer; fat is each of the human body demands (well, to some huge extent). For that dieter what this means is less muscle loss than what's possible on some diet. Be sensible?

As an added bonus, ketones yield just seven calories per gram. This can be higher compared to equal mass of sugar but less (22 percent (in reality) compared to the 9 calorie g of fat from whence it came. We enjoy metabolic inefficiencies similar to this. They mean we could eat more however, your human body will not obtain the calories.

Much sexier is this ketones can't be turned back in to essential fatty acids; your system excretes any excess from the pee! Speaking of that, there'll be a real little bit of pee; the shed in muscular glycogen, very low nourishment and very low aldosterone all equal massive excretion of extracellular fluid. For people which way hard, defined muscularity and quick, observable outcomes.

Seeing energy, our brain actually really enjoys ketones therefore we are apt to feel fantastic in ketosis - clean led, positive and alert. And as there's never a lack of fat to furnish ketones energy is elevated constantly. Usually you sleep and wake up feeling fuller once in ketosis.

Doing it right

From what's mentioned above you may realize that to enter ketosis:

Carbohydrate ingestion ought to be postponed; zero!

Protein ingestion should maintain low - 25 percent of calories in some max

Fat should account to get 75 percent + of carbs

With reduced insulin (as a result of zero carbohydrates) and carbs in the slightest, or below care, the dietary fat can't be deposited into adrenal cells. The low-ish protein usually means gluconeogenesis will immediately establish inadequate to keep blood sugar and, even perhaps your system enjoys it or not, there's all of the fat to burn up.

And burn it does. The high-fat is oxidized for cellular energy from the standard manner but winds up generating amounts of acetyl-coA that transcend the potential for the TCA cycle. The most substantial effect is ketogenesis - absorption of ketones from the surplus acetylcoa. In more specific terms: that the high fat ingestion "compels "ketosis up on your system. This is the way its own 'done '.

You simply need to throw away what you thought was true regarding carbs. Primarily, fat will not "make you obese ". The majority of the info concerning the evils of fats, specifically, is indeed intense or plain wrong any way; onto a ketogenic diet it's doubly inapplicable. Fatty foods create ketosis fly. And don "t stress; your heart is going to soon be a lot better than nice as well as also your own insulin sensitivity won't be paid down (there is certainly not any insulin round to start with)!

Once in ketosis it's perhaps not necessary, publicly speaking, to keep up absolute zero carbohydrates or low carbs. Nonetheless, it's still better if you'd like to reap the best rewards. In any case, supposing you're working hard, you are going to still desire to adhere to a cyclic ketogenic diet where you're able to eat all of your own carbs, fresh fruit and anything else, every 12 weeks, any way (more about this in the following article).

Do not be confused; 'done ' will not create ketogenic dieting fun or easy to your own culinary acrobats one of you. They're possibly the most restrictive diets that you may utilize and maybe not a choice if you never love monster solutions. Get out of your supplements almanac and workout an 20:0:80 proteincarb:dietplan. Yeah, its boring. For example, your author's everyday ketogenic diet plan is 3100 calories in 25:0.5:74.5 from just this:

- 10 xxl whole eggs
- 160ml pure cream (40% fat)
- 400g mince (15 percent fat)
- 60ml flax seed oil
- 30g whey protein isolate

Supplementation?

There really are a range of supplements which help out with making ketogenic diet plans better. But lots of popular supplements are wasted. Here's a summary of the main kinds:

Chromium and ala, although not carbohydrates 'mimickers' as most assert, improve insulin sensitivity leading to reduced glucose levels, greater glucagon and also a quicker descent to deeper ketosis

Nourishment is really a little waste - in most, 30% might be consumed by the muscles which, with nourishment, may not be meaningfully 'volumised'.

HMB (in case it works) would/should be a superb nutritional supplement for minimizing the catabolic phase before ketosis is achieved

Tribulus is exemplary and has highly recommended since it hastens the greater testosterone output signal of an ketogenic diet

Carnitine in l or acetyl-l form can be a almost important nutritional supplement for ketogenic diet plans. Lcarnitine is vital for the creation of ketones from the liver.

Glutamine, free form crucial and branched chain aminos are rewarding for pre and post training. Simply do not overlook the glutamine since it affirms gluconeogenesis

ECA pile fat burners are extremely beneficial and crucial though don "t be worried about the addition of HCA

Flax seed oil is a good but don't believe you want 50 percent of your calories out of fatty acids that are essential. 1 10 percent of calories will be more than adequate.

Whey-protein is optional - that you never desire an excessive amount of protein remember

A soluble fiber nutritional supplement that's non-carbohydrate established is good. But walnuts tend to be somewhat easier. Ketogenic diet plans offer you a lot of unique benefits that can't be ignored in the event you're pursuing the ultimate, very low body fat figure or body. But they're maybe not the most easy to use of any 'middle earth' undermine you might want will probably be the hardest of worlds. Your decision would be always to complete them not all.

The keto diet and fat loss

If you've had a want to lose a few additional pounds, and perhaps you may have encounter ketogenic dietplan, that is popularly called keto dietplan. It's a favorite weight reduction program which promises substantial weight reduction in a quick moment.

However way from what the majority of men and women believe it to be the diet isn't just a magic tool for weight loss reduction. Exactly as with any other nutritional supplement, it requires some time, needs plenty of modification and tracking to observe effects.

What's the keto diet?

The keto diet plan is geared toward placing the own body in ketosis. This diet regime is usually low-carb with higher intake of healthful carbohydrates, veggies and fats that are adequate. From this diet, there's also an emphasis on avoiding packaged sugars and foods.

You will find several sorts of keto diet plans: standard ketogenic, cyclical, concentrated and also the high-protein food diets. The gap in these depends upon the carbohydrate intake. The conventional ketogenic diet is low carb, higher fat and sufficient nourishment would be the very advocated.

Is your keto diet safe?

Most critics of all that the keto diet say it isn't safe due to the increased exposure of consuming high fat information. That really is directed by the misconception which carbohydrates are harmful to you. To the other hand, healthy fats are now very great for you personally.

With this particular diet, you obtain a lot of fats from sources such as nuts, avocado, fish, legumes, eggs, olive oil, palm seeds, oil such as chia and red meat.

Just how can the keto diet assist in weight reduction?

Just how can the keto diet work and help the system lose pounds? After to a higher carb diet, the body utilizes glucose from sugars and carbohydrates into fuel activities. When to a ketogenic diet, then you furnish your system using nominal levels of sugars and carbs.

With decreased sugars and carbohydrates provide, the sugar levels within the human body are depleted inducing the human body to search for different energy sources. Your system consequently turns to stored carbs to energy that's the reason why the keto diet contributes to weight loss.

This illness where the own body burns carbs for energy aside from carbohydrates is known as ketosis. Whenever the system goes into ketosis, it produced ketones since the gas supply as opposed to according to sugar. Ketones and sugar are the sole two power sources which fuel your brain.

Advantages of ketosis and also the keto diet

Besides only helping in weight reduction, putting your system in ketosis includes additional health benefits in addition. Here are a number of these:

- Enriched psychological clarity

- Enriched physical energy

- Steady blood sugar levels that causes it to be a fantastic cure for epilepsy and diabetes

- Enriched and improved skin tones

- Lower cholesterol amounts

- Hormone regulation particularly in women

The ketogenic diet is just one of the greatest food diets you are able to follow along with fat loss and also to enhance your general wellbeing. The diet may be utilized for kids that weigh too much. There are many studies which encourage that the dietary plan demonstrating substantial effects particularly when combined together with exe

Keto dieting? Here are 10 foods you have to have on your own kitchen

The ketogenic diet is a really successful weight reduction program. It uses high fat and lower carb components so as to burn fat rather than glucose. Lots of men and women are knowledgeable about this Atkins diet, however, the keto plan limits carbohydrates a lot more.

Because we're surrounded by junk food restaurants and processed meals, it's rather a struggle to steer clear of carb-rich food items, however, proper preparation could help.

Plan menus and snacks at the very least a week beforehand, and that means that you are not captured with just large carbohydrate meal choices. Research keto recipes on the web; you will find a number of very good ones to select from. Immerse yourself at the keto way of life, find your favorite recipes, and stay to them.

There really are several items which are principles of a keto dietplan. Make sure you get these products available:

Eggs - used at omelets, quiches (yes, significant lotion is legal on keto!) , hard-boiled as a bite, low carb pizza crust, and much more; should you prefer eggs, then you have a fantastic likelihood of success with this diet

Bacon – can I would like reasons? Broccoli, cherry garnish, legumes topper, blt's (no bread naturally; here is another blt at a bowl, then pitched in mayo)

Cream-cheese - lots of meals, pizza crusts, main dishes and desserts

Shredded cheese - pour taco meat in a bowl, then built in to tortilla chips from the microwave, microwave toppers, low-fat pizza along with enchiladas

A great deal of romaine and lettuce - fill upon the green vegetables; have plenty available to get a fast salad if food cravings struck

Ez-sweetz liquid sweetener - utilize a few drops as opposed to sugar this artificial sweetener has become the easiest and easiest to use that I have found

Cauliflower - frozen or fresh luggage you can consume this skillet alone, tossed in olive oil and roasted, mashed in imitation potatoes, chopped/shredded and utilized in area of rice beneath principal dishes, in low fat and keto pizza crusts, also even more

Frozen chicken tenders - consume a massive bag on hand; thaw fast and grill, saute, mix with top and veggies with garlic sauce at a low-carb flat bread, utilize within chicken piccata, chicken Alfredo, tacos, enchiladas, Indian steak poultry, and much more

Ground-beef - make a large burger and shirt with a variety of items from cheese, into sautéed mushrooms to grilled onions... Or cook and bake together with taco seasoning and then apply provolone cheese taco shells; toss at a dish with avocado, lettuce, cheese and sour cream to get a tortilla-less taco salad

Almonds (plain or roasted) - these really are a tasty and nutritious snack; nevertheless, make sure you rely on them since you eat, as the carbohydrates do mount up. Flavors contain habanero, coconut, vinegar and salt and much more.

The keto program is a flexible and intriguing means to shed weight, with a lot of yummy food options. Maintain these 10 things carried on your refrigerator freezer and larder, and you're going to be prepared to throw together some yummy keto snacks and meals at an instant's notice.

The ketogenic diet is a balanced solution for everybody who would like to shed weight. Stop by the healthy keto internet site, a very important resource at which keto dieters may get meal thoughts and keto diet truth.

Can be the keto diet clean or dirty?

In cross-fit diet recommendations we now have composed broadly about a fantastic diet for athletes. If you abide by a more keto style dietplan, or stick into some paleo regime, you will find good techniques and bad ways to complete it. A name does not clarify a certain diet method. It's possible to follow you into the correspondence, however in the event the foods you're using are of low quality, then you might well be doing more damage than good. Within this article we'll concentrate on the ketogenic (keto) daily diet plan.

A keto diet plan is defined as eating at a sense for the human body to create ketones. Ketones are made by the liver and this process is caused by ingestion hardly any carbohydrates and also a fair quantity of protein. The ketones can be employed by your body to get energy. Ergo a keto diet essentially burns up fat as your body's way to obtain fuel. The fat is burnt nonstop from the physique. Whenever the body produces ketones, it moves in to a state of ketosis. The ketosis will burn up fat before fretting about flaxseed. In other words, provided that you continue eating a ketogenic diet plan.

This attracts me to our subject of a sterile versus a cluttered keto diet. As this kind of diet plan is limited in carbs, an ordinary staple may be fish, meat, along with low-fat lettuce. It won't indicate it's nice to eat a fast food hamburger or alternative commercially raised meat. If you're just simply cutting off your carbohydrate intake, then you're living a "dirty "keto dietplan. The veggies, meat, fish, etc... , ought to be organic and non gmo.

We counsel you to avoid any processed food items or people packed with additives. These is going to do injury to some dietary plan and also keep you from living a poison daily life. Any dietary plan works better once the foods are clean and basic.

A keto diet includes a detoxifying procedure when consumed precisely. If you put in poisons throughout the foods, then you aren't helping your liver, or even your wellbeing.

Eat new, organic veggies. Attempt to eat an assortment of colored veggies high in fiber. The longer you do so, the more and better tasty they could taste. Provided that your own body will literally crave them to every meal.

So far as fat products, select healthful sources. These can be organic flax seed, coconut oil, salmon, or coconut oil. A number of them are deemed non inflammatory foods. Spicy foods are such as milk products or any of those nightshade veggies.

While alive the sterile keto diet, don't forget to stay hydrated. Lots of do not understand that water helps each one the everyday functions including organ and digestion production.

In closure, bear in mind, if you're alive the "dirty "keto diet, then you're doing a disservice. Stay 'wash "and keep healthier.

CHAPTER THREE

DOES A KETO DIET HELP LOWER GLUCOSE LEVELS?

Can be just a ketogenic diet protected for those that have gotten a diagnosis of diabetes? The foodstuff advocated for those who have higher blood sugar levels promotes fat reduction: a ketogenic diet contains high levels of fat and can be low in carbohydrates, therefore it's mysterious how this kind of high-fat diet is definitely an solution for relieving elevated blood glucose levels

The ketogenic diet underlines a minimal consumption of carbs and increased ingestion of protein and fat. Your body then reduces fat via a process known as "ketosis, " and produces a supply of gas called ketones. Usually, the diet improves blood glucose sugar levels while decreasing your human body's demand for insulin. The dietary plan was initially developed for epilepsy therapy, however the forms of food and also the ingestion regimen that it high lights, are increasingly being studied for its sake of people with diabetes.

The ketogenic diet comprises foods such as for example...

- Pasta,

- Fruits, and

- Bread

As a supply of body power. People who have diabetes suffer with shaky and high glucose levels, and also the keto diet helps them allowing your body to keep their blood glucose at a lesser healthier level.

How can a keto diet aid many with diabetes? In 2016the journal of obesity and eating disorders released an overview indicating a keto diet can help individuals who have diabetes by improving their a1c test outcome, significantly more than the usual dietplan.

The ketogenic diet puts focus on the ingestion of protein and fat, which makes you feel less hungry and consequently resulting in fat reduction. Protein and fat take longer to digest than carbohydrates plus helps keep up energy levels.

In short that the ketogenic diet...

- Reduce blood sugar,

- Enhances insulin sensitivity and

- Promotes less dependence on medications.

The keto diet plan. Ketogenic diet plans are somewhat strict, however should stuck to properly they are able to offer a healthful and healthy nourishment pattern. It's all about staying apart from carbohydrate foods inclined to spike glucose.

People who have type 2 diabetes tend to be counseled to concentrate with this particular diet because it is made up of mixture of low carbohydrate foods, including high quality content material, and medium protein. It's also crucial since it averts high-processed food items and indulges in processed and healthful foods.

A ketogenic diet should contain these kinds of food...

Low-carb veggies: eat veggies with each meal. Keep away from starchy veggies such as tomatoes and corn.

Eggs: they contain a very low quantity of carbs and therefore are a top source of nourishment.

Meats: consume oily meats but prevent excessive quantities. High levels of nourishment and low carbs may cause the liver turning protein to sugar, hence evoking somebody to turn out of ketosis.

Fish: an great source of protein.

Eat from healthful sources of fat such as seeds, avocados, seeds, and coconut oil.

Conclusion. Additionally, it is effective to really go by what the human own body requires in the place of that which you believe you want. Always follow your physician's advice about medications and nutrition and also consult him prior to starting a brand new diet program.

Even though managing your disorder can be quite hard, type2 diabetes isn't really a condition you must simply live with. You may make simple modifications to your everyday routine and lower your entire body weight and your glucose. Hang in there, the longer you can do it, the easier it gets.

Diabetes and fat loss - the differences between keto and paleo diet plans

Fat competitions smoking because the primary cause of preventable death. 1 reason is that the striking growth within the diabetes hazard frequently accompanying weight reduction. Thus, are you really currently interested in establishing a fresh diet regime, you aimed to not just assist you to drop weight but to restrain your blood glucose? You likely are looking for the most useful options out there. The two you'll come around since they truly are cool in the current times would be the ketogenic diet plan and also the paleodiet plan. Lots of men and women actually become confused between those while they really do are similar therefore that it can be difficult to differentiate between these.

Let's compare so that you may determine which is ideal for one...

Carb resources. To begin with, let us discuss carbohydrate sources since it is the point where both diet plans vastly disagree...

With the paleo diet program, your carbohydrate sources are likely to be some fruit, together with sweet potatoes. Together, you may very quickly reach 100 g or more of carbs between both of these foods.

The keto diet, alternatively, your sole carbohydrate origin is leafy greens, and also people are not restricted.

None of those many important differences between your ketogenic diet plan and also the paleodiet regime is that the ketogenic diet is deficient in carbs whereas the paleo isn't. You're able to produce the paleodiet really low carbohydrate if you'd like, however it isn't default. There was more flexibility in food choices.

Calorie counting. We return to calorie counting. Additionally, this is a location where both diet plans differ greatly.

With the keto diet, you're going to be macro and calorie counting quite significantly. You want to reach certain goals...

30% complete protein ingestion,

5 percent carb ingestion and

65% fat ingestion.

In case you don't reach these goals, you're not likely to proceed in to the "condition of ketosis, "that will be the whole purpose with this diet regime.

With the paleo daily diet, there are no strict rules about that particular. At the same time that you're able to count calories if you'd like, you usually do not need to. Evidently, your weight loss results will probably be better in case you really do track calories into a level since calories don't dictate if you gain or shed excess fat, however it isn't crucial.

Exercise fuel availability. That brings us to your second point - exercise fuel accessibility. In order have the ability to exercise with strength, you want carbs in your daily diet program. You can't get fuel accessibility in the event that you aren't wanting to eat carbohydrate-rich foods that means that the keto diet isn't going to encourage drastic physical exercise sessions. Because of this, the keto diet won't be optimal for a lot of people. Exercise can be an essential component of staying healthy, therefore it's advisable that you exercise and also don't adhere to an eating plan that restricts exercise.

Obviously, you may perform the targeted ketogenic diet regime and also perhaps the cyclic ketogenic diet plan, both of that are you containing carbohydrates from the diet in a certain time...

The targeted ketogenic diet offers you eating carbs before starting your fitness session whilst

The cyclic ketogenic diet requires that you eat a bigger dose of carbohydrates over the week end, and that can be intended to keep you throughout the remainder of the week.

Should you follow either of them, you may decide on any carbs you need; nevertheless, it generally does not need to need to be merely sweet fruit or potatoes.

There you've a few essential differences between both of these approaches...

The ketogenic diet is just only one focusing more about tracking macros and it is meant to help with weight loss whilst

The paleo diet concentrates longer about good food choices and health insurance and expects fat loss comes as a outcome.

Even though managing diabetes might be very hard, it isn't really a state you must only live together with. Make simple adjustments to your everyday routine - comprise exercise to reduce your glucose and your own weight.

Ketogenic diet plans for running diabetes

Ketogenic diet plans will be used since 19-24 in pediatrics as remedy for epilepsy. Even a ketogenic (keto) diet is the one that's full of fat and low in carbohydrates. The plan of this ketogenic diet will be really to changes your body's metabolic fuel by burning carbs to fats. With the keto diet, then the human body metabolizes fat, in the place of glucose into energy. Ketones are a portion of this procedure.

Through the years, ketogenic diet plans are used to deal with diabetes. 1 rationale was that it soothes diabetes in its real cause from reducing carbohydrate ingestion resulting in lower blood glucose, which in turn, reduces the demand for insulin that reduces insulin resistance and associated metabolic syndrome. This manner, a ketogenic diet can improve blood sugar (glucose) levels while at the exact same time diminishing the demand for the insulin. This standpoint gift ideas keto diet plans as a far healthier and more efficient plan than simply injecting sugar to counter act the usage of foods that are high.

A keto diet plan is actually an extremely restrictive diet plan. From the timeless keto diet as an instance, one has got about 80 per cent of caloric requirements from fat and 20 per cent from carbohydrates and proteins. This really is a noticeable departure from the standard where your system operates on energy out of glucose based on carbohydrate digestion however by seriously restricting carbs that your body is made to make use of fat alternatively.

A ketogenic diet necessitates healthy food ingestion from fats that are beneficial, such as olive oil, grass-pastured legumes, organic leafy greens, avocado, fish like salmon, cottage cheese, avocado, almond butter and raw nuts (raw pecans and macadamia). People on ketogenic diet plans avoid all pasta, pasta, potatoes, wheat, pasta, starchy veggies, and milk. The diet is lower in vitamins, minerals, and nutrition and require nourishment.

Low carb diet is often suggested if you have type two diabetes because carbs turn into blood glucose that in huge amounts cause blood sugar levels to spike. Ergo, to get a parasitic who has elevated blood glucose, eating additional glucose is similar to courting danger. By changing the attention of sugar, some patients may experience blood glucose.

Altering the human body's primary energy source of carbs to fat results in the byproduct of fat metabolism, ketones from blood circulation. For some diabetics, this may be dangerous being an accumulation of ketones could cause a risk for developing diabetic ketoacidosis (dka). DKA can be a health emergency requiring the help of doctor. DKA signs include always large blood sugar levels, dry skin, polyuria, nausea, and breath with a fruit-like odor and breathing difficulties. Infection may lead to diabetic coma

Diabetes - if you work with a ketogenic diet regime?

As somebody who is working hard to restrain or protect against diabetes, 1 diet you could have found out about is your ketogenic or keto diet program. This diet can be just a rather low carbohydrate diet regime composed of approximately...

5 percent complete carbohydrates,

30 percent protein, and a

Whopping 65 percent dietary fat.

If there's one thing that this diet is going to do, its particular help control your glucose. That being said, there's more to eating well than simply controlling your blood glucose levels.

Let us discuss a number of the chief reasons this particular diet does not always pile up to be great as it sounds...

Inch. You will be lacking soluble fiber. The first major issue with the ketogenic diet is that'll be lacking in fiber. Just about all veggies have been cut using the plan of action (independent of the exact lowcarb varieties) fruits and vegetables are not permitted. High fiber cereals are out of this equation, which this leaves one with primarily fats and protein - 2 foods containing no fiber in any way.

Proceed with this diet plan and you're going to find you begin to feel backed up in virtually no time.

2. You're going to be low in energy. Yet another large issue with the ketogenic diet is that'll be reduced in energy to perform your exercise regime. Your own system can only use sugar as a fuel source for very acute exercise also in the event that you're not ingesting carbohydrates, then you will not have any sugar available.

Consequently, that the ketogenic diet isn't appropriate for everyone who wishes to lead a busy life style with routine work out routines.

3. You can suffer brain fog. People who are employing the ketogenic diet can also notice they suffer with brain fog. Again, that is as a result of this truth that your brain chiefly conducts glucose off.

Some individuals may find after having a couple weeks of utilizing the diet that they begin to feel like their brain can switchover to using ketone bodies like a fuel supply, but the others might never see they start to feel a lot better.

Overall, this diet just cannot benefit a few individuals with this reason.

4. Your antioxidant status will decline. In the end, the previous difficulty with the ketogenic diet is a result of the deficiency of vegetable and fruit material - the antioxidant status will sharply diminish.

Anti-oxidants are very important to fending off free radical damage, therefore this is simply not something to take lightly. If you are not carrying them you might wind up ill later on.

Therefore keep these points in your mind as the dietary plan has some risks. The ketogenic diet arouses fat rather than sugar. It was initially created as remedy for epilepsy however today the impacts of the dietary plan have been looked in to help type2 diabetics lower their blood glucose sugarlevels. Ensure that you discuss the dietary plan with your health care provider prior to making any dietary modifications.

Even though managing your disorder can be quite hard, type2 diabetes isn't really a condition you must simply live with. You may make simple modifications to your everyday routine and lower your entire body weight and your glucose. Hang in there, the longer you can do it, the easier it gets.

Lowcarb and keto diet junk food menu choices: the way to eat immediately at restaurants

For all those who eat low-fat or keto food diets, there's more often than not something you'll be able to eat at every fast food restaurant or place. Plan ahead. Before entering a restaurant, then have a look at their menu and nutrition advice on the web in your home or even together with your cell mobile. It is usually great to understand the safe options before being enticed by menu items which you have to not have on a lowcarb dietplan.

In order to create it simpler to locate a fast keto-friendly option, I have compiled a set of several restaurants and take out places along with people items which I have found are the cheapest carbohydrate (& most emotionally pleasing) choices. These aren't all ideal alternatives, however when you are stuck using no additional choices thanks to location or time limitations, they'll do at a pinch.

It is a enormous assistance that fast-food places are needed to create nutrient content. It makes simpler to adhere to the keto plan daily. The carbohydrate count I am list is approximate and can be net g.

Generally, there's often a salad option anywhere you're. In burger joints, only take out the bun, and lots of places provide lettuce packs alternatively. Chicken should not have breading.

Just as a complication, it will help to possess a fork and knife handy on your car or handbag. Big, juicy hamburgers in miniature parts of lettuce wind upon the desk or on your own lap. Small, flimsy fast-food plastic ware additionally causes eating. Pullout of your very own hardy utensils and love!

Now for your meals choices... Below are several pretty obvious basic principles to follow:

- Forget the bun or wrap

- Forget the pasta, potatorice

Salads - no croutons. Stay to low-carb options - caesar, blue cheese, ranch, chipotle. Have a look at the name that might provide you a hint, matters such as "honey " from the honey Dijon or even "sweet " from the dressing table name - those usually are not just a great selection. Check the fixing for things which can be high in carbohydrate content.

Steak - pick grilled or sautéed. Avoid any poultry that's breaded.

McDonald's - elect for any hamburger (zero gram) or broiled chicken (2 gram) minus the bun and topped with cheese, mayo, mustard, onions, etc.).) no more ketchup. Insert a side salad (3g). The caesar salad with grilled chicken or perhaps the bacon ranch salad with broiled chicken are 9g.

Burger king - same beans advice as McDonald's: hamburger (zero gram) with no bun and topped with cheese, mayo, mustard, onions, etc.).) no more ketchup. The tender grill chicken sandwich minus the bun is 3g. Beware - it might seem the veggie burger is not low, however it really is 19g of carbohydrates therefore that is about the complete day of carbohydrates on keto. Insert a side salad (3g). Even the tender grill chicken garden salad is 8g without dressing or croutons. The tender crisp poultry salad isn't feasible. Don't attempt.

Bonus - dessert!?! - That the brand new apple chips aren't fried and therefore are 5g net carbohydrates without caramel sauce.

Subway - probably should bypass subway when possible. Even the buns and wraps are typical high in carbohydrates. I figure you might only ask them to throw the ingredients at a wrapper sans bun, but it will not seem appealing. I don't have any advice on which the carbohydrate count is for each bun-less sub, however you could probably find out it - grain or pepperoni is nice, but can be "sweet onion " poultry fine? Whatever idea. Stick into the cakes, however, realize you are going to just receive iceberg lettuce (4g).

Carl's junior and Hardees - this series supplies "lettuce wraps "- your hamburger wrapped in a sizable parcel of lettuce for easy low-carb intake. (as I have said I tried it and also do not think it's great. Allow me to take my fork rather) bun-less options - six buck hamburger (7g), 1/2 thick-burger (5g), charbroiled chicken club sandwich (7g/10g in Hardees). Grilled chicken salad without croutons is 10g. Negative salad is 3g.

Jimmy john's - even the unwich - a sandwich wrapped in lettuce - fits the bill. Meats are nice, just ensure that the ingredients aren't carb-rich.

Wendy's - you can attain your beans at a lettuce wrap or perhaps a box. Any hamburger with lettuce. Mayo contains corn syrup, also it is 1g. The chicken dish noodle is just 1 gram. It might be arranged at the poultry club sandwich or even the greatest chicken noodle sandwich. Best fries: chicken Caesar (7g), blt poultry salad with broiled chicken. Negative salads aer 6 g or 2-g to get caesar.

Pizza hut and other pizza areas - it's likely to get accustomed to eating pizza without any crust. You want to consume twice as much, however if there exists a celebration or dinner outside you cannot stop in a pizza place, simply slip the cheesy toppings away and eat the massive messy pile of toppings and cheese. Aside salad is really a wonderful addition. Otherwise, simply elect in making pizza acquainted with a lowcarb crust.

Mongolian barbecue - yes! Bunch your bowl with fish, poultry, onion pieces, and mushrooms, then high with the black bean sauce. I understand beans have carbohydrates, yet this sauce tag says inch g of carbohydrates per oz (each sauce is more apparently labeled). Insert a little bit of garlic and await that griller to perform his job out. It goes without mentioning that you bypass the beers, tortillas rice. Request the wait staff never to attract them into the dining table.

Italian restaurants - all these require a little cute, nevertheless they could be more conquered! A few ideas: just how about chicken masala within an

Italian location? Make certain that it can't arrive with rice. Substitute broccoli or any other keto-friendly side-dish or perhaps a massive salad. Chicken piccata can be an opportunity.

Mexican and Chinese restaurants would be the most challenging, as any low carbohydrate choice really isn't the reason why to visit the restaurant at the very first location. In a Mexican restaurant, then that I often tend to find yourself a massive burrito without a beans and also disperse the tender tortilla out such as a plate. Eat the internal components and then throw the tortilla.

If you need to go to some Chinese buffet (I attended a dinner in one), it is possible to discover options, and however they probably are not planning to become your beloved general tso's. Think about the salad bar choices? Eggs? The insides of egg rolls, and that I ate the insides just of crab rangoons. Regrettably these notions leave a significant heap of discarded cubes and heavy fried outside bits in your own plate also causes it to look as if you truly waste food.

Wings everywhere - standard beef sauce is generally ok in addition to garlic parmesan

Convenience stores might be very good alternative, too! 7 11 has packs of hardboiled beans, cheese cubes, slim jims, almonds, and pork rinds. Pork rinds arrive in an barbecue flavor plus they truly are zero carbohydrates.

Bear in mind, what you may decide on, contain the bread, potatoes, noodles, rice, chips, and tortillas. And be careful for the potential for cornstarch, breadcrumbs, and different additives. With good preparation and a fantastic attitude, it is possible to discover nutritious keto and low-fat options when dining outside, and follow your successful keto diet program.

The ketogenic diet is a balanced solution for everybody who would like to shed weight. Stop by the healthy keto internet site, a very important resource at which keto dieters may get meal thoughts and keto diet truth.

Moving keto: exactly why that it is great for you

Keto diet plans have come on strong at the last year 5 and also for justification. It's really a excellent solution to not just lose those unwanted pounds fast, but but also a wonderful method to have strong and stay that way. For the ones which have tried the keto diet and so are still about it, then it's over only a diet program. It's really a method of life, an entirely new way of life. However, just like any significant shift in our own lives it's not a straightforward person, it can take an unbelievable amount of dedication and dedication.

Beneficial to a few although perhaps not for everybody? - though a ketogenic diet was used to substantially improve people's wellbeing, you will find several out there who really do not talk about the majority's manner of believing. However, is this exactly? From the time we can remember we're educated that the only real means to eliminate this additional burden was supposed to stop eating the fat packed foods which we are accustomed to eating daily. So instructing visitors to eat healthful fats (the crucial word is healthy) that you can simply understand why a few folks are doubtful concerning why and how you'd eat more fat to attain weight reduction and reach it fast. This theory goes contrary to what we have known about weight reduction.

The way keto launched - launched by endocrinologist roll-in woodyatt at 1921 when he discovered the 3 water -soluble substances aceture, b-hydroxybutyrate and acetoacetate (known as ketone bodies) were created by the liver as a consequence of starvation or in the event the individual accompanied by a diet rich in higher fat and low carbohydrates. Later on this year per guy from the mayo clinic by the name of russel wilder called it the "ketogenic diet regime, "and used it to deal with epilepsy in small kids having fantastic success. But due to advancements in medicine it had been substituted.

My struggles starting keto –I first started keto, I'd made an effort at the keto diet before about roughly a few weeks before but was unable to create it during the initial week. The very first week keto is that the most peculiar portion of the complete procedure, this really is once the dreaded keto flu looks additionally referred to as the carbohydrate flu. The keto flu can be an all pure reaction that your body experiences when changing from burning sugar (glucose) as a result of burning fat as an alternative. Lots of men and women who've gone about the keto diet say it feels like withdrawing from a addictive chemical. This will last anywhere between 3 days into a whole week, this just lasted a day or two in my personal case.

Individuals that have'd the keto flu record feeling tired, achy, nauseous, dizzy and also have dreadful migraines among anything else. The first week is when people attempting a keto diet neglect and cease, remember this happens to everybody else in the method of course, in the event that you're able to get beyond the very first week that the hardest part has ended. There are certainly a couple remedies you need to utilize to assist you cope with this demanding spell. Accepting electrolyte supplements, staying hydrated, drinking bone broth, eating more beef and getting lots of sleep. Keto flu can be a unfortunate event that does occur to everybody else as your entire body expels the normal diet. You merely need to power through.

What exactly does a ketogenic diet appear to be? - if the average man eats meals full of carbohydrates, their entire body chooses the ones carbohydrates and converts them to sugar. Glucose is your body's key source of gas when carbohydrates are found in the human anatomy, onto a keto diet are very low in case any carbs consumed that compels your body to use different kinds of energy to maintain your system functioning correctly. This is really where healthy fats get involved, with the lack of carbohydrates the liver carries essential fatty acids in your human body and transforms them to ketone bodies.

A perfect keto diet should contain:

- 70 80 percent fat

- 20 25% protein

- 5 10 percent carbohydrates

You shouldn't be eating over 20g of carbohydrates daily to keep up the normal ketogenic dietplan. Personally, I ate significantly less than 10g each day for an even more extreme experience but that I achieved my first targets and then some. I lost 28 pounds. At only a bit under 3 weeks.

What's ketosis? - if your system has been compromised completely by fat it passes a condition referred to as "ketosis, " that will be an all pure condition to your own human anatomy. Once each one the sugars and also unhealthy fats are taken out of the body throughout the first two or three weeks, the human body is currently free run on healthy fats. Ketosis has lots of potential benefits-related to accelerated body weight loss, performance or health. In some specific instances such as type1 diabetes excess ketosis can grow to be excessively dangerous, in which in some specific cases paired together with intermittent fasting might be immensely good for individuals affected by type two diabetes. Substantial work will be conducted with this subject from Dr. Jason fung m.d. (nephrologist) of this intensive dietary administration program.

Everything I may and cannot eat for some one brand new to keto it might be very hard to abide by a lowcarb diet, though fat may be your basis with the diet you shouldn't be eating all sorts of fat. Healthy fats are very essential, however what's healthy fat you may possibly ask. Healthy fats could contain sweet meats, (poultry, goat, beef, venison), wild caught fish and fish, pastured pork & poultry. Eggs and salt-free butters may be ingested. Make sure you avoid starchy veggies, fruit, vegetables, and grains. Processed food items really are on no account accepted in virtually any form or form in the ketogenic diet program, artificial milk and sweeteners may also pose a severe matter.

CHAPTER FOUR

THE KETOGENIC DIET: A MORE DEPENDENT FACTOR ON FAT-BURNING

When utilizing a ketogenic diet program, the body gets more of a fat burner compared to the usual carbohydrate-dependent machine. Several studies have connected with the consumption of increased levels of carbs to evolution of several disorders like diabetes and insulin resistance.

By character, carbohydrates may be absorbable and can also be be readily kept by your own body. Digestion of carbs starts from the moment that you put them in orally.

After you begin chewing them amylase (the enzymes which consume carbohydrate) on your spit is at the job behaving to the carbohydrate-containing food.

At the gut, carbohydrates are further broken. If they put in to the small intestines, then they are subsequently absorbed into the blood. On becoming into the blood, carbs generally boost the blood glucose level.

This increase in blood glucose level arouses the instantaneous release of insulin to the blood. The more complicated the growth in blood glucose, the greater the total amount of insulin that's re lease.

Insulin is a hormone which leads to excess glucose in the blood to be removed as a way to lessen the blood glucose level. Insulin carries the carbohydrate and sugar you eat and stores these as glycogen in muscle cells or as fat from adipose tissue to future utilization as energy.

Nevertheless, that the body can create what's called insulin resistance if it's always confronted with such high levels of sugar in the blood. This scenario might easily bring about obesity as your body has a tendency to immediately save any surplus sum of glucose. Health issues like diabetes and cardio vascular disease may also lead in this illness.

Keto diet plans really are low in carbohydrate and high in fat and also are correlated with improving and reducing several health issues.

Certainly one of those foremost matters that a ketogenic diet is to stabilize your sugar levels and restore lepton signaling. Reduced levels of insulin in the blood let you feel fuller for a extended time frame also to own fewer cravings.

Medical advantages of ketogenic diet plans

The program and execution of this ketogenic diet has enlarged significantly. Keto diet plans in many cases are signaled as a member of this procedure solution in numerous health ailments.

Epilepsy

That really is ostensibly the principal reason behind this maturation of the ketogenic diet plan. For some cause, the metabolic pace of epileptic seizures reduces if patients have been set on a keto dietplan.

Pediatric epileptic cases would be the most receptive to this keto diet. There are kids who've experience seizure removal after a couple of years of working with a keto dietplan.

Kids with epilepsy are usually predicted to fast to get a couple of days prior to beginning the ketogenic diet as part of the treatment.

Cancer

Research suggests the therapeutic effectiveness of the ketogenic diet plans against tumor growth might be enhanced if coupled with certain medication and procedures under a "press-pulse "paradigm.

It's additionally promising to be aware that ketogenic diet plans induce the cancer-cell right into remission. Which usually means that keto food diets "starves cancer "to lower the indicators.

Alzheimer infection

You will find several signs that the memory acts of patients with Alzheimer's disease grow after taking advantage of a ketogenic diet plan.

Ketones are a fantastic supply of alternative energy to mental performance specially if it has been resistant to insulin. Ketones also supply substrates (cholesterol) which help to correct damaged membranes and nerves. These helps improve memory and cognition in Alzheimer's patients.

Diabetes

It's usually consented that carbs are the principal culprit in diabetes. Accordingly, by simply lessening the level of ingested carbohydrate using a ketogenic diet, then you will find increased opportunities of improved blood glucose control.

Additionally, mixing a keto diet along with additional diabetes treatment plans could somewhat boost their general efficacy.

Gluten allergy

Many people with gluten allergies are curable for this specific illness. But, after having a ketogenic diet revealed improvement in related ailments such as digestive distress and bloating.

Many carbohydrate-rich foods are full of gluten free. So, using a keto diet, then a great deal of the gluten ingestion is reduced to the absolute minimum as a result of removal of a massive assortment of carbs.

Weight reduction

That can be possibly the very typical "deliberate "use of the ketogenic diet now. It's established a niche for itself from the Egyptian dieting tendency. Keto diet plans also have been part of many dieting regime because of its well-recognized complication of helping weight reduction.

Though originally maligned by most, the expanding number of beneficial body weight loss results has helped the ketogenic to raise adopted because of a significant weightless program.

Form aforementioned health advantages, ketogenic diet plans additionally supply a few overall health benefits including these.

Increased insulin sensitivity

That really is obviously the very first goal of a ketogenic diet plan. It is helpful you to stabilize your glucose levels consequently improving fat burning off.

Muscle preservation

Since nourishment is oxidized, it will help to preserve lean muscle mass. Losing muscle tissue induces someone's metabolic rate to decrease since muscles are ordinarily very metabolic. Employing a keto diet helps preserve muscle tissue while the body burns off fat.

Controlled ph and respiratory function

A ketoc food plan helps to reduce lactate consequently improving both ph and respiratory functioning. A condition of ketosis so will help keep blood glucose ph in a wholesome level.

Increased immune system

Employing a ketogenic diet will help fight aging anti-oxidants while also reducing inflammation of the intestine consequently helping your immune system stronger.

Paid off allergic levels

Consuming fewer carbohydrates even though you're to the keto diet may help reduce blood glucose levels. That is a result of the rise in condition of lipolysis. This also contributes to a decrease in ldl cholesterol levels and a rise in hdl cholesterol levels.

Reduced appetite and cravings

Adopting a ketogenic diet enables one to lessen your entire cravings and appetite for calorie foods that are rich. As you commence eating healthy, satisfying, and healthful highfat food items, your appetite opinions will naturally begin decreasing.

The sideeffects of working with a ketogenic diet for fat loss

The ketogenic diet, colloquially referred to as the keto dietis a favorite diet containing high levels of carbs, sufficient protein and very low carbohydrate. It's likewise known as a low carb-high fat (lchf) diet and a very low carbohydrate dietplan.

Ketogenic diet plans are intended to induce your system to access a condition known as ketosis. Your system generally uses carbohydrate as its principal supply of energy. This owes to the point that carbs would be the easiest for your body to consume.

But should the body operate out of carbs, it adheres to using of protein and fats for its own energy production.

Ketosis effectively changes the system's natural formula from burning sugar to rather begin burning off fat as fuel. This change of their human body's metabolic process might include some potential negative effects as your body attempts to correct it working out.

Shifting to the ketogenic diet isn't so an easy task to accommodate to notably at the very first onset. But, bear in mind that these unwanted side effects are temporary. More than a few of them are able to endure for a day or two while others can last for weeks.

So you need to devote your self-time, both emotionally and emotionally, to effortlessly produce the switch.

While creating the switch into some ketogenic diet plan, you can find just two physiological changes which you could experience. All these would be the keto influenza and keto breath.

Keto flu

That can be just one thing that anybody starting a ketogenic diet needs to prop around. It's a requirement in that you go through a number of those various unwanted effects which can come along with having a ketogenic diet plan.

Keto influenza is often seen as an light headedness or brain fogginess, nausea, headaches, stomach aches, and muscular soreness. You can also experience increased feelings of irritability, depression and trouble concentrating.

Interestingly, all of these are common signs of the flu, and thus the name. All these signs are temporary and maybe not everybody else working with a ketogenic is influenced by these.

These signs are usually brought on by the glucose withdrawal occasioned by the reduced carbohydrate ingestion. Additionally, an imbalance in the own body electrolytes like magnesium, calcium, magnesium, and sodium may affect the way the system responds to the consequence of an ketogenic diet plan.

Keto breath

You will find just two possible reasons set forth people on ketogenic diet plans experience this strange breath difficulty.

Your system will not not shop ketones and ergo they have to be excreted from your system. Ketones may be excreted via the urine as acetoacetate.

They can be excreted via the breath inform of acetone. And so that the further ketones you make, the more the further acetone you pass through your own breath. Regrettably, this could induce unpleasant-smelling breath once with a ketogenic diet plan.

On another hand, greater protein intake may also bring about keto breath. That is due to the fact that the method by which in which the human body digest fats and fats is quite various. The digestion of fats usually produces ammonia that your body excretes throughout the pee.

Nevertheless, that the greater ingestion of carbohydrates may possibly end in the indigestible levels staying on your gut system also gets fermentation. This produces ammonia that's then discharged throughout your breath.

Keto breath may last for approximately a week to just under per month. It mostly depends upon how well the body adjusts to ketosis.

Micro-nutrient deficiencies

This will result from the rigorous restrictions on carbohydrate ingestion. A whole lot of carbohydrate-rich foods are both full of minerals and vitamins.

The acute restriction on carbohydrate intake could consequently cause deficiencies in a few vital nutritional elements. For that reason, we ought to not merely be dedicated to the micro-nutrient counting concerning proteins, fat, and carbs but also needs to don't forget the mineral and vitamin micro nutrient contents too.

That can be why nutritional supplements are largely advocated when applying a ketogenic diet plan. Supplementation helps augment any micro nutrient imbalance which may occur when applying a ketogenic diet plan.

What's the very best diet for losing weight and fat?

We've got all heard about these fad diet plans such as the carrot diet and also perhaps the apple dietplan. I will be here to inform you food diets which work. Most those food diets include fad, crash, and "dumb "food diets. A true diet comprises a mixture of muscle building protein, energy satisfying carbohydrates, and healthful fats for the heart.

For shedding weight, ketosis could be your ideal diet and isn't just a fad. In an keto diet, an individual could eat a lot of fats and protein along with little carbs to make it happen human body at a condition of ketosis. As there's absolutely not any longer glycogen in the entire body, by the shortage of carbs, the system will build ketone bodies out of the own fat cells to fuel the body and the human mind. Provided that you're eating enough protein, you are going to sustain your muscle and lose excess pounds of fat easily.

Becoming in to ketosis takes approximately 37 days based upon your own present storage. Ketosis feels strange in the beginning because you're going to undoubtedly be lethargic and might experience headaches as well as nausea. But these symptoms proceed a way. Additionally you will shed a lot of weight initially as a result of water.

Normal foods on a keto diet comprise nuts, whey protein, eggs, sausage, bacon, coconut oil, poultry, legumes, and so forth; whatever which comprises a large quantity of fats and protein and also no carbohydrates. A vitamin nutritional supplement can be drawn at a keto diet as you cannot eat vegetables that are much. (Nevertheless you can consume a minimum of one bowl of salad)

It requires powerful will power to keep on keto since in the event that you cheat eat or once something awful your own body will probably be from ketosis. A procedure that required 37 days today must be re done.

In a nutshell, keto is your finest short-term diet that you can do to cuttingedge.

The ketogenic diet - ultimate weight loss diet

The keto dietplan. What's the keto diet? Essentially it's whenever you deceive the system to using your bodyfat as it has main power source in the place of carbs. Even the keto diet is popular way of fat loss fast and economically.

The science behind it

To receive your own body to a ketogenic condition you need to eat a high fat diet plan and affordable protein using no carbohydrates or almost no. The percentage should be approximately 80 percent fat and 20% protein. This will definitely the rule for the initial two weeks. Once in a ketogenic condition you'll need to maximize protein intake and decreased fat, then percentage will probably be approximately 65 percent fat, 30 percent protein and 5 percent carbohydrates. Protein has been raised to spare muscle tissues. Whenever the own body intakes carbs it induces an insulin spike that means that the pancreas releases insulin (helps save bile, proteins and excess calories as fat) therefore ordinary sense informs us if we expel carbohydrates then a insulin won't store excess calories as fat. Perfect.

Now your own body has no carbohydrates as an energy-source your own body needs to locate a fresh source. Fat. This works out perfectly in the event that you would like to shed excess fat loss. Your system will breakdown your system fat and put it to use as energy rather than of carbohydrates. This condition is known as ketosis. This really is the condition you would like the own body to function as in, makes sense if you'd like to shed excess fat while maintaining muscle mass.

Now to the diet program part and just how to organize it. You will have to ingestion no less than a g of protein each day pounds of lean mass.. This will help in the healing and repair of muscle tissues after such and workouts. Bear in mind the ratio? 65 percent obese and 30 percent protein. Well should you weight 150 lbs of lean mass that means 150g of protein every day. X 4 (level of calories a g of protein) which is 600 calories. The rest of your own calories should come from fat. In case your caloric upkeep is 3000 you need to consume around 500 less that may indicate that in the event you'll need 2500 calories each day, approximately 1-900 calories has to come out of carbohydrates! You have to consume fats to fuel the human system that in yield may even burn body fat! That's the principle of this particular diet, you need to consume fats! The benefit to ingesting dietary fats and also the keto diet is you may not really feel hungry. Fat digestion is very slow that functions to your benefit and aids you are feeling 'full'.

You may end up doing so Monday - Friday after which "carb-up " over this weekend. After your final work out on Friday that really is as soon as the carbohydrate up begins. You have to ingestion a liquid carbohydrate together side your whey shake post workout. This helps to create an insulin spike and also helps to get the nourishment that your body urgently needs for muscle growth and repair and also refill glycogen stores. In this period (consuming) eat exactly what you need - bread, noodles, crisps, ice-cream. Such a thing. This is going to be helpful for you since it is going to re fuel the own body for the upcoming week in addition to restoring the body's nutritional supplement requirements. Once Sunday starts back its straight back into the no carbohydrate high fat medium diet. Keeping the system in ketosis and burning off fat as energy may be an excellent solution.

Still another advantage to ketosis is your gain in their condition of ketosis and burn the fat that you 'body is going to likely be depleted of carbohydrates. As soon as you bunch with carbohydrates you'll appear as complete as (without body fat !)) Which can be fantastic for these events on weekends once you attend the shore or parties!

Now allows recap on diet.

-must input the condition of ketosis through the elimination of carbohydrates in the diet whilst in-taking high-fat moderate/low protein.

-must ingestion fiber of a type to maintain your plumbing as clear as if you know exactly what I am talking.

-after in ketosis protein consumption has to be that of a gram of protein per pound of lean mass.

-this is fairly much it! It will take devotion to no eat carbohydrates through the week out for a great deal of foods consuming carbohydrates, but don't forget you'll soon be rewarded greatly for the own dedication. You shouldn't remain static in their condition of ketosis weeks end since it's dangerous and are likely to wind up getting the own body embracing make use of protein as a gas supply that's no. Hope it has helped and decent chance dieting!

Supplementation for cyclical ketogenic dieting

Keto dieting is tremendously effective for helping people to lose excess weight loss. But in the event that you're using ckd - or your cyclical ketogenic diet - then you're likely to need to incorporate several basic supplements so as to keep your muscle mass, then ease the fatburning process, and maintain your wellbeing in that stressful time period.

Creatine is just one nutritional supplement that's remarkably effective even though found at a low carbohydrate, higher protein atmosphere. Supplemental insulin retains the insulin amounts of one's own body marginally raised, which compels your own muscle tissues to put up an addition quantity of plain water. This also contributes to bigger, fuller and rounder muscles that are effective at transferring weight from your fitness center. As time passes, the extra movement equates to muscle - in a ketogenic atmosphere! Therefore maintain your nourishment dosage moving - 10 g every day should suffice. You should absolutely continue to relish the exact beneficial character of Creatine.

The eca stack, or a mixture of 25 mg ephedrine, 200 mg caffeine, and 250 mg ibuprofen can be often used throughout a ckd diet as a way to reduce some body-fat by simply exposing numerous procedures in your system. ECA increases your body temperature slightly. Appetite continues to be curbed. Magnesium is encouraged. Users typically find their abdominals soda out and veins become observable with each passing day. Toss in the essence of this keto diet, having its lost fat and water, and there is a recipe to get fat burning victory! Eca ought to be properly used 3 days, one day away for optimal results and in order to prevent dependence to this caffeine.

Maintain a really close attention up on your pee color and odor if employing this specific supplementation and diet. The own body will probably be under a fantastic deal of stress - your own kidneys particularly! For those who have any history of kidney disorders, or you've abused supplements previously, the combo of those ketogenic supplements and dieting might not be perfect for you personally.

If you're utilizing ketogenic dieting, so you ought to be consuming a good deal of water daily - around two gallons! Every one of the 3 above facets - keto dieting, nourishment, and eca supplementation require another quantity of water daily out your everyday requirements.

You ought to always consult your doctor before plunging to a ketogenic diet regime. Completing a blood, as you'd before running a steroid cycle, can also be an excellent idea. This really isn't your normal diet in which you shave just a tiny fat off your everyday ingestion and lose a couple of pounds. Ketogenic dieting can be utilized by the very best professionals from the whole world to realize great contour - and may be utilized by you personally - for as long when you diet and nutritional supplements attentively.

Ketogenic diet plans - recognizing ketosis and ketones

The ketogenic diet, colloquially referred to as the keto diet is a favorite diet containing high levels of carbs, sufficient protein and very low carbohydrate. It's likewise known as a low carb-high fat (lchf) diet and a very low carbohydrate dietplan.

Ketogenic diet plans are essentially built to cause a state of ketosis within your system. After the quantity of sugar within your system gets too low, your system switches into fat instead of an alternate source of energy.

Your human body has two principal gas sources that are:

- Sugar

- Free fatty acids (ffa) and, to some lesser degree, ketones created from ffa

Fat residues are stored within the shape of triglycerides. They truly are usually broken into long-chain essential fatty acids and glycerol. Shut-off the glycerol in the adrenal molecule permits the discharge of those 3 free fatty acid (ffa) molecules to the blood to be applied as energy.

The glycerol molecule enters the liver at which three molecules of it unite to create 1 glucose receptor. For that reason, as the own body burns off fat, in addition, it produces glucose for a byproduct. This sugar enables you to fuel pieces of the brain in addition to some other pieces of the human anatomy which can't run using ffa.

But while glucose may travel through the blood by itself, triglycerides and cholesterol require a carrier to maneuver from the blood. Cholesterol and triglycerides have been packed at a carrier referred to as sub-par lipoprotein, or ldl. Ergo, the more substantial the ldl particle, the more the more greater triglycerides it comprises.

The entire means of reducing off fat deposits because of energy produces carbon dioxide, oxygen, and chemicals called ketones.

Ketones are produced by the liver from fatty acids that are free. There are made up of two categories of atoms linked with way of a carbonyl functional set.

Your human body doesn't have power to put away ketones and for that reason they need to be used or shut. Your human body excrete them through the breath because acetone or by means of the pee as acetoacetate.

Ketones could be used by human body cells as a source of energy. Additionally, the mind are able to take advantage of ketones in generating approximately 70-75percent of its own energy condition.

Like alcohol, ketones simply take priority for a gas supply over carbs. This suggests when they have been saturated from the blood, they has to be burnt before sugar can be applied as a fuel.

What causes ketosis

After you begin eating less quantities of carbs, the system receives smaller source of sugar to utilize as energy in contrast to earlier.

The reduction in the total sum of absorbed fats and also the next decline in the sum of available sugar, slowly forces your entire body to move in their condition of ketosis. Ergo, the entire body moves into a state of ketosis whenever there isn't sufficient number of sugar available to your own human body cells.

Starvation induced ketosis

Fasting and starvation conditions usually demand no or reduced ingestion of food which your human body is able to consume and convert to sugar. While starvation can be involuntary, flaxseed is really a more mindful choice you create to deliberately not consume.

Nevertheless, that the body enters into a "starvation mode " once you're sleeping, once you skip dinner or when you go to an easy. The deficiency of food ingestion causes a decrease in blood sugar levels. Because of this, your system starts to break it down glycogen (stored sugar) stores such as energy.

The nourishment is converted into glucose and used as energy in the human body. Within this condition, the human body starts to burn up its stored fats. Ergo, the creation of ketone bodies (ketogenesis) is triggered by a deficiency of glucose that is available.

Whenever that the level of ketones in blood interrupts the molecules of sugar, your human body tissues will begin using their ketones because their supply of energy.

I get requested about ketogenic diet plans to get bodybuilding or weight loss goals much. Individuals always desires to learn what he most useful diet is what they are able to do in order to shed weight faster. Truthfully, many people don't have any idea what they're getting themselves in to.

While a ketogenic diet can work then a low-carb diet, "Ireally don't understand if people are prepared for them.

To start, a ketogenic diet plan is one where there aren't any carbohydrates. Without carbs your system turn to burn up fat as the main fuel supply. As that really is happening your human body is able to tap in to stored body fat for energy and also we can wind up thinner. Well while that's potential we will need to check at what could happen.

To begin with your own energy is going to be emptied. Without carbs the system wont understand what energy source to turn to for a couple of days and that means that you will experience feelings of fatigue at the same time you train or before the entire body becomes accommodated at using fatloss. While this is not a poor thing that you must know you have to improve your practice intensity. There is absolutely no way you can keep training with superb high volume at the same time you utilize these diet plans.

The following thing that you must realize about having a ketogenic diet for weight loss or bodybuilding is just you want to consume more protein then ordinary. As you never have carbohydrates, and carbs are protein you want to take more protein therefore that you never shed muscle tissues. Therefore ensure you are eating at the very least 6 meals each day having a portions of nourishment coming daily.

Then you must make certain you are receiving enough fiber. Try to absorb fiber from several sources like vegetables and fiber powder or nutritional supplements such as physillum husk. Nowadays you have to bring some supplements as you ought to be certain you do what you can to burn up fat onto those keto food diets to weight loss and muscle building supplements. To begin with, make certain that you consume healthy fats such as omega3 fish oils, cla, and gla. These fats can assist you burn more bodyfat. Then you definitely would like to buy a fantastic branch chain amino acid powder because bcaa's help retain muscle tissue and protect against muscle breakdown.

Therefore in conclusion, a ketogenic diet might be the most appropriate for fat loss or bodybuilding nevertheless, you want to be certain that you are eating enough and carrying in the ideal nutrition or you'll lose a lot of muscles.

Keto and lowcarb recipe thoughts: 5 delicious pizzas for both lowcarb and keto dieters

You can nevertheless eat pizza to the keto diet program, however, it requires a little imagination. If dining out, I order a thin-crust pizza, then choose my fork and then slip each of the toppings from the crust. It is helpful to arrange a pizza with a great deal of toppings. Ordering one topping onto a heavy dish leaves one very little left to eat.

Like most food choices on keto, the very best pizza would be that the main one that you create yourself. Try out the low carb pizza soup recipe, then utilize a number of those suggestions for toppings:

- Mexican pizza - use either conventional (low-fat) sausage sauce or enchilada sauce and top with taco-seasoned ground poultry or beef. Insert a little bit of salsa, sliced onions, sliced jalapeno peppers, along with some spicy sauce (taco bell hot sauce would be the smallest in carbohydrates). For a few extra flavor, add chopped onions. Along with chopped avocado following baking.

- Greek pizza - sauce, feta cheese, red onions, olives, and also what about a few artichoke hearts?

- Buffalo poultry pizza - thatIhad been thrilled to realize frank's exotic steak wing sauce is low in carbohydrates. If you prefer spicy, sexy, sexy, utilize chopped fried poultry, a few blossoms, crumbled blue cheese, and also the skillet sauce to generate a zesty pizza. Do not forget to scatter a tiny blue cheese dressing outrageous.

- Indian pizza - there exists a neighborhood restaurant near which focuses primarily on Indian championships that gave me the notion of earning my very own. In the event you decide to produce this yummy choice, then you may work with a packed Indian food recipe for poultry in addition to the lowcarb crust and then add a few vegetables. If you would like to begin from scratch up some poultry with traditional Indian spices, just for example masala, curry powder, carrot, and also any other hot Indian noodle you may consider. Add vegetables if desirable.

- Alfredo pizza - make use of a keto diet-friendly Alfredo sauce or only spoon a few outside of a jar. Top with fish or poultry, also carrot, garlic, roma tomatoes - and also extra parmesan cheese if you would like.

Obviously, you could have every one of the conventional pizza options:

Meat fans - pepperoni, sausage, bacon, pork, anything you want. All these are extremely lowcarb choices

Veggie fans - mushrooms, tomatoes, onions, all sorts of peppers, artichoke hearts... You mention it, it is going to taste great.

Three (or four, or 2) cheese - attempt feta cheese, blue cheese, goat cheese, cream cheese or every different tangy cheese, also to -- or instead -- of those conventional shredded mozzarella. (recall, many lowcarb crusts will also be made from cheese. You might wish to be mindful of it)

As soon as you have a good lowcarb crust, the topping some ideas are endless. Keto dieters have a lot of alternatives. The only real limitation is the own imagination.

The ketogenic diet is a balanced solution for everybody who would like to shed weight. Stop by the healthy keto internet site, a very important resource at which keto dieters may get meal thoughts and keto diet truth.

CHAPTER FIVE

VEGAN DIET

The vegan diet is well regarded for health benefits, and particularly - weight reduction. Lots of people have experienced the vegan diet to its only purpose to shed weight and have succeeded in doing this. If you're trying to find a healthful and secure diet to shed weight, and also are thinking of the vegan diet, then you want to think about: is it really safe? Might it be wise? Can it be sustainable?

Could it be safe?

If you experience the vegan diet at a sensible, well-orchestrated fashion, it is possible to be certain it is both secure and healthier. You want to make certain you're eating various different foods each single day to make sure you are receiving optimum nourishment - but you have to get this done to almost any diet program. In the event that you should resort to eating vegetarian processed foods frequently, your quality of life would clearly suffer.

Vegan crap food comprises packet crisps, sexy chips, dairy-free candy and chocolate bars, so-called 'health-bars' which can be packaged with sugar etc.. In the event that you should take foods like this on an everyday basis and eat them as opposed to one's meals that are proper, you're damaging the human body. As an alternative, it is possible to elect to create your own personal vegan baking snacks like dairy-free, low-sugar snacks, brownies, cakes, breads, oat and nut pieces, etc., including dates, dried fruits, fruits and veggies, nuts, olive oil, extra virgin coconut seeds and oil. Undergo your diet plan at a timely and sensible manner, and provide the body the nourishment it needs.

Might it be wise?

If you have to shed excess weight, the vegetarian diet is in fact one of those nutritious food diets which you are able to embrace to achieve that. It's unwise to elect for a fad diet that's saturated in fat, saturated in nutrition and also leaves you feeling fuller. It's possible to enjoy avocadoes, coconut oil, seeds and nuts within this particular diet - like most wreck diet plans now. It is also possible to enjoy a variety of gourmet, healthful cooking therefore that you won't have to feel dizzy. By creating your own flavorful and wholesome vegan baking soda recipes, you're ensuring you will continue being joyful and articles with this particular diet, as opposed to miserable and cranky.

Thus, if the vegan diet supplies you with a lot of healthful nourishment, gives the body adequate healthful fats and doesn't leave you feeling deprived, do you mention it is wise or unwise to go down this pathway? I'd say it is wise.

Can it be sustainable?

There are lots of longterm vegans that are on the vegan diet their whole lifetime or for centuries. These individuals are almost always slender and slender and possess a healthier, luminous complexion and a zest for life which the majority are jealous of. Unlike crash diet plans, this particular diet is more still sustainable. Why? You won't feel deprived since there are lots of yummy alternatives to eat. You are able to enjoy a broad selection of amazing vegetarian recipes or dinner recipes that are simple to locate in novels, on the web, or out of vegan recipe e books. Medical advantages of this diet is likely to cause you to recognize it is well-worth forsaking dairy and meat products. Many did and are continuing to do this now. Is this you?

Weight reduction on the vegetarian diet is safe, sustainable and wise. Therefore perhaps it's now that the opportunity to throw off all your crash diet thoughts and ideas, and elect for a healthy, vegetarian lifestyle which may leave the entire body, spirit and mind joyful, healthy and well-nurtured.

The anti-aging aftereffects of the vegan diet

A lot of people in the-world mock people on the vegetarian diet, however, men such as these needs to really be pitied. Why? Soon, they will develop some individual medical problems and you will be seeking an eating plan to help them recover their health and live more. And the better way to save their health compared to embracing veganism! Why don't we find out.

Which will be the health benefits of the vegetarian dietplan?

Anti-aging

A plant-based diet was famous for hundreds of years due to its anti-again consequences. People who eat mostly or mainly foods that are fermented will survive more than dairy and meat eaters. This was demonstrated. A u.s study-based on half-a-million people demonstrated that drinkers of processed and red meats expired more usually prematurely than men who ate a more dietplan. The evidence is that there folks! Most vegans are still a mature old age, nor develop diseases or disorders that strike the remaining portion of the people. Yes, anti-ageing is among the very most well-reported health and fitness benefits of the vegetarian dietplan!

Beauty

Only look at anette larkinsa famed vegan woman who's over 70 yrs of age but looks a day over the age of 40! Additionally google mimi kirk - that can be in her own mid-seventies but looks much younger. Then there is dan mcdonalda vegan raw foodist who's within his mid-forties. His smooth, luminous skin looks like this of a boy! Additionally, consider portia de rossi, alicia Silverstone, anne Hathaway, Michelle Pfeiffer and Natalie Portman. These magnificent beauties are known to adhere to along with diet, and also their perfect skin and luminous faces attest into it! It's been reported that individuals who embrace veganism have undergone a unscrambling of skin conditions like psoriasis and psoriasis. Young skin is certainly a portion of this healthy vegetarian diet!

Reduce danger of cardiovascular disease, diabetes, cancer, rheumatoid arthritis symptoms, and hypertension

Studies suggest that a routine use of animal protein and fats increases a individual's risk of developing chronic illness including diabetes, cancer, cardiovascular disease, rheumatoid arthritis and hypertension. Studies also demonstrate that men who eradicate dairy and meat products out of their diet and replace them using foods that are wholesome, legumes, whole grains and soy will lessen their probability of developing those diseases, and also eradicate or reduce those. By way of instance, it's been demonstrated that men that have early stage prostate cancer may reverse or stop the development of the cancer should they embrace a vegetarian diet plan and also expel all dairy and meat food. Yes, the healthier vegetarian diet is famous for decades due to its amazing healing capacities and remarkable wellness advantages.

The vegan diet offers many amazing health benefits that have been demonstrated again and again. Many men who've embraced veganism won't offer this up, as the health benefits are just too precious to concede!

Steps from the transition to your vegan diet: the best way to begin a vegan diet

For all those who are fresh to the diet, the considered unexpectedly abstaining out of all dairy and meat food can be utterly frightening. In the present society, many folk comprise beef, eggs and legumes into a sizable proportion of these daily food ingestion. Ergo, if it's your own desire to embrace the diet and you're inundated at the thought of leaving supporting your favorite foods immediately, you should alternatively make a slow transition into the dietplan. The next 8 steps describe the way to begin a vegetarian diet with victory!

The gradual transition for your beginner vegan:

Measure 1: expel red-meat

Step one should be rather simple. Cutout all lamb, steak, poultry and other red meat in the dietplan, but still let yourself eat white meat (poultry, fish and fish). Also bear in mind you could find meat-free "bacon " and vegetarian "mince " from many supermarkets and health stores. Whenever you're beginning to really feel comfortable never wanting to eat red meat, then go on into another point.

Measure two: expel chicken

Simply eat fish and fish products for a time period, and give a wide berth to the rest of the meats including poultry. Become accustomed to preparing meals with meat, and get started researching recipe ideas for vegetarian meals.

Measure 3: expel fish & seafood

By today you may be going entirely vegetarian. Rather than eating beef and fish, your own protein will probably be arriving from beans (chick peas, lentils, black beans etc.), whole grains, tofu, vegetarian "patties, " vegetarian "mince, " along with other meat-free goods like vegan "bacon " bear in mind that now it's possible to find yourself a great deal of vegetarian foods at the supermarket. Get to understand the services and products and brands offered. In addition, you shouldn't be terrified of kale, it might be immensely versatile and flavorful if cooked correctly. It has got the capability to absorb the flavors of other spices and foods it is cooked/marinated together, so discover the way you can cook it so that it is going to taste yummy!

Measure 4: expel cheese

That really is the first phase of the transition from vegetarian to vegan. For the newcomer vegan, the idea of abandoning cheese products may seem to be quite down-heartening, since lots of folk like cheese on daily basis: in the lunch, inside their own cakes, in their sandwiches, even within their noodles... The list continues! But if you'd like to finally benefit from the countless excellent health benefits of the vegetarian diet you must expel cheese from the daily diet plan. If that is problematic for you (almost certainly), then purchase several of the mock-cheeses (vegan) from the regional shop)

Measure 5: expel eggs

This is also a difficult thing for a lot of, but you should be conscious that eggs are a creature product, and so giving up them is essential for anyone that want to carry to the diet. It's possible to create lots of yummy tasting egg dishes using peas (e.g.: to-fu "scrambled eggs "), of course in the event that you abide by a excellent recipe and receive the tastes right - you most likely wont actually miss out your eggs!

Measure 6: expel cream & butter

You have now eliminated all of your solid animal foods in the dietplan. The upcoming recommended point on your transition into vegetarian would be always to deteriorate out of cream and butter, and all services and products containing both of these ingredients. It's possible to use a number of different fats and oils alternatively such as coconut oil, coconut oil, and vegan margarine. You might need to cook the majority of one's daily life candies today, as most snacks and cakes at stores and cafes comprise eggs and butter.

Measure 7: expel milk

This should not be too difficult, as there are lots of vegetarian choices to milk in these times. You're able to drink soymilk, rice , almond milk, etc.. You are able to bake or cook with all these nutritious milks, eat them together with your cereal, or even drink them by the glass!

Measure 8: get some good vegan recipes

Now you are 100% vegetarian, and all your foods from today on will probably likely be vegetarian, you want to collect a great deal of yummy vegan recipes! You can find some fantastic recipes on the internet on websites, sites, or even simply by buying an expert vegan recipe e book. Your recipe collection ought to include a wide selection of recipes, including vegetarian foods, lunches, dinners, sandwiches, sandwiches, breads, noodles, desserts and fast meals.

The vegan lifestyle is equally rewarding and challenging at the exact same moment. Those not used to the vegetarian diet needs to possess a thorough knowledge and comprehension of this life style so create the transition into becoming vegetarian as simple as you possibly can. This will make certain you may know precisely what to expect, and certainly will allow you to deal with and have an understanding of some challenges that might appear. The next 3 hints are particularly for the newcomer vegan. They'll allow one understand how to begin a vegetarian diet successfully. To put it differently, the way to guarantee smooth sailing!

Hint # 1 - know in-advance the rewards & suggestions

The rewarding facet of this vegetarian diet requires the remarkable health and emotional benefits including weight reduction, clean skin, fewer allergies, and a change or decrease of chronic disease, diminished aging approach, inner calmness and endurance, and also capacity to concentrate and focus. The difficult facet involves how relatives members and friends will respond originally and longterm, the cravings that the you'll grow (particularly at the onset of diet to the newcomer noodle), the struggle of eating dinner out, initial detoxification symptoms, and also feeling as a small weight when people needs to prepare distinct food only for you personally.

Research additional individuals who've gone to the vegan diet plan also and determine what they've undergone. What exactly did they say is the hardest aspect? Can it make easier to them? Additionally discover exactly what advantages and disadvantages that they have experienced. You'll see in the research that a lot of folk will concur that the rewards undoubtedly outweigh any challenges or barriers experienced within the vegan way of life!

Hint no 2 - find & collect great vegan recipes

This really is among the most significant suggestions to adhering to this dietplan. It's critical for every novice vegetarian to begin their diet fully prepared, i.e., together with lots of rice recipes. Possessing a significant number of recipes accumulated will ensure the following:

Inch. That one may prepare something fast & easy once you're feeling tired or busy

2. Could save you the aggravation of having to seek out vegan recipes whenever you're not really in the mood.

3. When you're urge a candy treat, you're able to goto a own recipe set and bake your own healthier cake or piece, in the place of going off your diet plan or eating package noodle crap food.

Locate your vegan recipes online through web sites, blogs, you tube, or simply by buying a vegetarian recipe e book (be aware: vegetarian recipe e books comprise tonnes of yummy recipes made from professional vegetarian chefs). Otherwise, you might buy a vegetarian recipe cook book in the community book store, however normally, this is the most costly choice. The option of where you buy your meals is yours.

Hint no 3 - let family, friends & coworkers know

It's vital to notify buddies, family members and even coworkers which you're embracing a vegetarian life. This will function as a protection for you and can to make your transition into the vegetarian diet as stress-free as achievable. How so? Listed below are a couple of situations that you'll be guarded from:

Inch. When buddies or family to see you personally, they know that you're eating vegan-only food, also will keep from bringing biscuits or snacks you cannot eat. In reality, they are going to more than likely have gone to the problem of choosing the vegan cure by the supermarket - only to talk with you personally!

2. You may end up saved from plenty of questions and interrogations in restaurants and cafes, because friends and family have been completely advised your final decision (as well as to a big extent, your own interrogation will be over!!!)

3. In societal parties, end of year parties, and parties, it's very likely that the sponsor will probably guarantee there is certainly some food there you are able to eat. There is nothing worse than visiting an event and being unable to eat some of their food (already been there, done this. I actually don't advise that you put yourself in this situation).

According to the vegan life is an incredibly rewarding travel - most longterm vegans can attest to the. If you're still wondering "why should I proceed vegan? "and "how does it benefit me personally? " this informative guide will allow you to realize that the huge benefits of the vegetarian diet really are infinite. In addition, it is going to allow you set realistic goals to to aid you in the transition into becoming vegetarian. Just don't forget a lifetime of good health and lots of blessings are going your path if you select to get this remarkable life style change.

The vegan transition: recommendations & help

Inch: note of the advantages of adopting the vegetarian diet program, and make note of or emotionally note which ones that you may love to realize. One of the very reported advantages of the vegetarian diet are as follows:

Weight reduction, clear skin (no psoriasis, psoriasis) glistening white eyes, healthful nails and hair, towering energy, inner calmness and bliss, ability to concentrate and attention, a new found zest forever, low fat but nutrient-dense super-foods, reduces cholesterol, prevents and reduces the signs of illness including cancer, and type two diabetes, higher blood pressure, arthritis, etc., loss or perhaps a whole unscrambling of allergies, allergies, headache, bad breath and body odor.

2: things do vegans eat? You want to locate out this as a way to proceed vegan.

In short, the vegetarian diet is made up of fruits, veggies, nutsseeds, whole grains, legumes, legumes, lentils, meat substitutes, avocado, coconut oil, olive oil, vegetarian smoothies, ham snacks (e.g.: crackers, brownies, cakes, pieces), fresh juices, cooked sauce, raw sauce, leafy vegetables, steak bread, pasta sandwiches and sandwiches, along with vegan soups. You may realize that all one of your favorite foods will probably possess a "vegan clone "recipe in these times. That is due to the rising prevalence of this dietplan.

3: obtain a great recipes

Do not be overly fearful of earning some recipes and meals with cream, meat, butter or cheese. There are all those mouthwatering vegetarian recipes today which are powerful in flavor and certainly will most likely taste a lot better compared to the non-vegan edition! It is possible to get various recipes on the web now, either on blogs and websites, or even simply by downloading a specialist vegetarian recipe e book. The recipe e books frequently have a huge selection of recipes to select from and therefore are manufactured by professional vegetarian chefs that understand just how to get vegan food taste and look great! You ought to collect various vegetarian meals, such as vegetarian breakfasts, lunches, dinners, salads, cakes, breads, muffins, pieces, chocolates, juices and smoothies, etc..

4: start away slowly.

It may be daunting for most folk to produce this type of significant life style change immediately. Therefore why don't you start by eating two or even three vegetarian foods each week. Whenever you're convinced for this, create the transition into eating a meal every day. Do lots of research "what do vegans eat "so you understand precisely what your vegetarian foods and recipes should include. As soon as you've been eating a vegetarian meal per day for quite a while, you're likely already beginning to notice some progress in your wellbeing, appearance and wellbeing. I encourage one to make another thing of one's daily life transition from eating just two vegan meals daily, and when you are able to, move mostly or even all vegan. This whole process might take months, weeks or possibly per year. You want to proceed at your own comfortable pace.

5: ditch that your bad customs

Should you carry on some your old bad habits on your vegan dietplan, your good outcome and health benefits will probably be greatly jeopardized. Reduce in your own caffeine and alcohol. Do not eat a lot "vegan unhealthy foods "for example ham packet fries, biscuits, chocolate bars, etc.. Enjoy these sometimes but not each single day if you would like to drop weight, tone up, clean your epidermis or find improvements in your own energy. Therefore kick against your old customs hard and then flush them down the toilet!

Why must I proceed vegan? You asked. The vegetarian diet delivers a large amount of amazing advantages, physically, mentally, emotionally and spiritually. You ought not let anything hold you back from discovering to yourself this gorgeous, low-carb diet. Create the vegan transition slow if you need to, however, stay focused, remember your own priorities, and always attempt to provide for your wellbeing insurance and wellbeing, regardless of what might come your way.

CHAPTER 6

VEGAN DIET AND ITS HEALTH BENEFITS

Few Americans know what a vegetarian diet is, or exactly what it may mean to your own wellness. Rather than a diet full of produce, the standard American diet is significant in animal grains, meats, and milk. In this method of eating has long been becoming worse with each creation. As it grows, so do lots of people's waistlines. Eating a vegetarian diet rather is just a healthful option. If you take in a vegetarian diet for a brief while, or keep for a life, veganism may be rewarding life style change.

Slim down, enjoy extra energy, and feel great by generating the switch into veganism.

Veganism is really a type of vegetarianism that's marginally more limited. While a vegetarian won't eat beef, a few still like eggs, milk, honey, and other animal products and solutions. Vegans, alternatively, avoid all animal products potential. Many avoid wearing wool and leather as these are animal merchandise. Vegans need to always be looking out for animal-based food additives. 1 common instance is red food dye that will be created of a sort of beetles.

Is veganism difficult to follow along with first glance, it seems quite tricky to adhere to a vegetarian dietplan. Animal items are anywhere, by the gelatin into chocolate. Many foods you wouldn't be prepared you'll possess animal solutions, do. In a few portions of the planet, opting to eat a vegetarian diet might be exceedingly hard to complete. But for a lot of people from the U.S. That there is certainly a plethora of food options once you learn the best places to appear. Health food stores and specialty shops tend to be somewhat more inclined to transport vegetarian food which grocery chains that are typical. Yet some much larger chains, such as Walmart, are starting to transport vegetarian and vegetarian alternatives.

Small, neighborhood grocery shops frequently have a fantastic choice of quick foodstuffs which are vegetarian friendly. Otherwise, they maybe more favorable towards making these options available to fulfill needs. When venturing out to eat, a few restaurants are much better suited to supplying vegetarian alternatives. Spanish, both south and central American, along with many Asian foods possess excellent vegetarian alternatives. And more vegetarian friendly restaurants have been opening across the country every day.

If necessary, you can constantly request the chef to put up the creature services and products for the own dish. Vegan snacks are simple to discover. Fresh produce, together with seeds and nuts, are all snacks which contain absolutely no animal products and solutions.

Try out a few of cashews, a good fresh fruit salad, along with perhaps a square of chocolate for an easy dish bite.

Can it be delicious?

You will find vegan dishes all over the earth, dishes which most people usually do not really realize are vegetarian. Hummus, fried okra, salads, chocolate. A great deal of items which people like on a regular basis don't have any animal products in any way.

Where the average American diet concentrates mainly on animal and meat fats, appearing out on our civilization we will get a broad range of yummy foods to savor. Whilst the demand grows, many food firms are currently offering vegetarian choices which are equally as yummy as the foods that they replace. From vegan variants of sausage, bacon, hamburgers, and ground beef, you'll find fantastic alternatives for folks thinking about a vegetarian diet program however, maybe not ready to say farewell to meat.

Vegans don't need to supply up their dessert options. Cakes, biscuits, ice creams, and much more can be made without eggs and milk, plus they're equally as yummy as the common versions. Try out a piece of curry apple pie, topped with dish ice cream produced from almond milk. Lots of men and women realize that since they conform to a vegetarian diet, their own awareness of preference no longer necessitates foods that are heavily cooked. Matters can taste candy with sugar before, which makes desserts a bit better.

As their strategies wash out the crap built-up, they are more sensitive to exactly what they eat.

Is veganism safe?

A balanced vegan diet could be incredible for the wellness. Obviously, the trick is keeping it more balanced. A diet of just vegetarian snacks, whilst vegan, would perhaps not be healthy in any way. Adhering with a balanced food plan and recalling to eat foods in moderation can allow you be fitter and shed weight. Even individuals who're at a wholesome weight range will probably feel a lot better if their entire body washes the creature services and products outside.

Common features of a longterm vegan

Thus a lot of people speak negatively of this vegan diet and this isn't any real surprise. They've now been led to trust their life time that eating milk and meat can allow one grow strong and fit, and thus should you not eat the foods that your quality of life are affected. But it is the wellness of milk and meat eaters that's affected, maybe not the other way round. This also contributes to this question: may be your vegan diet healthy all things considered?

To be able to answer this particular question, I've recorded below 5 shared features (whether psychological or physical) of a longterm vegetarian that I have noticed. All of them have these 5 beneficial faculties generally.

Inch. Skin care

A longterm vegetarian will possess excellent, flawless skin. Unlike milk and cheese eaters, they don't suffer migraines from ingesting an overconsumption of hard-to-digest milk product. Frequently vegans tend not to utilize make up, or hardly any, since their skin is so therefore good and also they don't have any flaws to cover up.

2. Hair

Vegans have healthy, luxury hair. The nutrition they are receiving out of their fruits, nuts, vegetables, legumes and whole grains are doing their own body wonders. By consuming their own body a wealth of nutrients that are essential, it's not surprising that their own hair and beauty look really remarkable. While the famous saying goes "you are what you consume " vegans live evidence with this expression.

3. Physique

Someone that has maintained the vegetarian diet for an elongated time period will just always be lean and slender. That is most likely largely as a result of the simple fact that they aren't wanting to eat any high quality, non-toxic dyes, lotions, butters as well as legumes. Together with their digestive-system in the ease, their own body has plainly functioned on shedding excess fat (when these were overweight in the first place), also isn't planning to place it straight back on anytime in the future. Once you find a vegan munching on an apple, or even a vegetable and bean salad you realize the reason why they're so slim!

4. Happiness

It can't go unnoticed that men on the vegetarian diet possess a deep zest for life, a passion and longing to escape bed and greet the day with a grin. Hand consistent with their abundant delights is that their incredible energy levels that baffle the regular person. How can an individual be vibrant, energized and happy? You wonder. The advantages of the vegetarian diet keep on getting better and better!

5. Health

Persons who've adopted veganism for an elongated time frame consuming excellent wellbeing, and rarely will need to go to the physician. They aren't over weight, they usually do not need high cholesterol, plus so they usually do not suffer with elevated blood pressure. Eating a diet in eating foods that were wholesome was reported to stop most ailments, including diabetes, together with a vast selection of other chronic disorders. A more life expectancy may be inserted into the list. The vegetarian diet is demonstrably a healthy person.

Is your vegan diet healthy? This may readily be replied after detecting the clear physiological and psychological wellbeing of a vegan. As the typical person is afflicted by ill-health, weight and fatigue issues - a vegetarian is booming, appearing the epitome of health, also has a zest for life that's envied by most. It appears that veganism may be your best way to really go after all.

Proof the vegan diet is worth pursuing

The Egyptian belief of veganism is the fact that it's dangerous, with a lack of nourishment, and also certainly will leave someone feeling deprived. Sadly, this couldn't be further away from the reality. If you're blessed to become more conversant with a longterm vegetarian, you are going to likely marvel in their slender and slender body, their perfect natural and skin splendor, and also their clear zest forever. May be your vegetarian diet healthful? Listed here are some just 5 famous health and fitness benefits of the vegetarian diet which are noticed again and again by men who embark with this life style.

Inch. Weight loss

Fat loss is among the very most well-reported added benefits of the vegan diet program. And minus the usage of greasy, calorie-laden dairy and meat food, this isn't any real surprise. Being an all natural low-carb diet regime, veganism can be definitely an perfect life style choice for men who want to drop some extra weightreduction.

2. Clean upward of skin issues

Since milk products like cheese, butter and cream are renowned for worsening psoriasis, eczema, eczema and other skin care conditions - and it's not any surprise that by removing those foods a individual's skin can heal or radically improve. Lots of people that have experienced the healthy vegetarian diet also have reported that a clear-up of these acne and also have observed that an overall healing in these skin.

3. Abundant energy

Heavy meats along with hard-to-digest cheeses and milk food will frequently leave an individual feeling lethargic and tired after being absorbed. This is exactly why many men and women feel tired and lacking energy. By minding those foods and replacing them with fresh veggies vegetables, legumes and lentils - it is possible to be sure your levels of energy will probably undoubtedly be steady daily. Therefore as opposed to feeling tired and tired once you get home from work in the day, you'll discover yourself desiring to really go for a night walk, or carrying your puppy for a walk as an alternative!

4. Zest for life

Lots of men and women who ditch dairy and meat food discover their depression and low moods have improved greatly. That is possible because frequently, a sick poorly-nourished human anatomy ends in a poor, very low soul. To the other hand, a wellfed, nutrient-dense diet ends in an optimistic, joyful state of mind. Vegans have been famous for their joyful mood and zest for life.

5. Prevents, treats, cures & alleviates health conditions.

Ditching dairy and meat food and substituting them with vegetables, fruits, seeds, nuts, wholegrains, legumes and lentils is an perfect choice to take care of many health and fitness diseases. The vegetarian diet is ideal for treating elevated cholesterol and higher blood pressure, preventing certain cancers, cardiovascular disease, diabetes and obesity as well as relieving a variety of ailments and pains like arthritis. All these are a few of many excellent health benefits of the vegetarian dietplan.

Is your vegan diet healthy? Whether this diet may prevent and cure chronic illness, ease fat loss, clean skin infections, provide excellent levels of energy, also empower an individual to nurture a zest to life - I'd absolutely say that the vegetarian diet is healthy. Cannot you agree? All these 5 health advantages demonstrate that veganism may be well worth pursuing.

Vegan observations

Whilst you're fighting together with your sicknesses allergies, lower levels of energy, inadequate skin and surplus pounds, your own vegan friend or work mate is booming and appearing slim and joyful. How is it? Just how can a man or woman who omits milk and meat from their diet looking so healthy? Maybe the vegetarian diet would be your solution following...

Is your vegan diet healthy?

The vast majority of folks may say no if asked "may be your vegan diet " that is likely predicated in the collected beliefs with the years pitched via the networking, novels, so nutrition experts, as well as supplementing relatives members and friends. A lot of people honestly feel that if an individual were to embrace a vegetarian way of life and eradicate dairy and meat products out of their diet, then they'd be lacking crucial minerals and nutrients in their diet especially protein. For that reason, their health are affected.

But wait a minute... You're person whose health is affected. You're the person who's afflicted by weight difficulties, lethargy, a scarcity of energy, a body and also a down trodden face. Along with the majority of one's own friends, family and work mates are experiencing bad health insurance and assorted human anatomy problems. Consequently need to agree you have to do something amiss.

If you're lucky enough to become more conversant with a few vegans that you will more than likely observe they have a lot of issues in common. To start with, a longterm vegetarian will always be lean. They won't be overweight. Second, a vegetarian routinely have a great deal of electricity and an evident zest for life. Paradoxically they are going to seem very healthy along with also their hair and skin is going to be of great illness. Fundamentally in the monitoring, you'll have ascertained that a vegetarian is healthy. The advantages of a vegetarian diet are demonstrably clear. For that reason, they need to do something right!

Advantages of a vegan diet

As you have probably observed that the vegan will probably be lean and slender, possess exemplary nourishment skin, strong and healthy hair, excellent levels of energy, are all creative, and also possess a passion forever. All these are merely a few of the visible advantages of the vegan diet program. There are clearly many different added benefits of veganism which you usually do not know of.

Various other perks of veganism comprise inner calmness and bliss, obtaining a joyful and easygoing vibe, no more longer digestive issues including bloating, flatulence and gut upsets (frequently due to milk and meat), also a solid purpose and attention in life, and also the sensation that you do something perfect for the body and mind.

Therefore, is your vegan diet healthy? From evidence and observation, the response will be yes. By the point of view of a closed mind and a blind eye, the solution is no. But after evaluating the and wellbeing of a vegan that is long-term - exactly what do you say?

Why are too many people going about your vegan diet?

You have only learned that a second of one's friends/workmates/acquaintances has embraced veganism. You're perplexed with their own decision, and also you don't have to wonder, 'could be your vegan diet ' 'can there be something they understand and that I really don't?' this might just be the situation. Lots of men and women do not know of the amazing curative benefits of the vegetarian diet program, and it isn't completely their fault. Why don't?

· health practitioners are not going to let you get rid of meat and milk products from the dietplan. They would like you to continue returning again to them. If you're well and healthy, they may miss out in your business.

· the tv/media isn't planning to widely promote the benefits of the vegetarian dietplan. Rather, they need their audience to gratify in cooking shows (together with dairy and meat displayed), supermarket dairy and meat ads, etc.). To put it differently, they don't really wish to end up losing their own audience.

· the milk industry is not going to inform you that a lot of individuals are allergic to eggs, milk and cheese. Doing this could be greatly detrimental for their prospective company.

· your parents are not going to let you proceed veganism. They'll stay to their widely held belief you have to drink milk daily for strong bones and eat red meat regularly for 'crucial protein' for healthy muscles.

So your beliefs on dairy and meat food are only a conglomeration of thoughts, beliefs and teachings out of the networking, health 'professionals," the dairy and meat business, along with well-meaning relatives.

What exactly is that the truth?

Is your vegan diet really healthy? Consider the next few tips, and then decide for yourself if embracing veganism could be your thing to do.

In accordance with a single U.S.-based study on approximately 120,000 individuals, drinkers of red meat have a substantially high level of dying.

Vegans consume no animal fat or cholesterol, so therefore, their odds of developing cardiovascular illness (which will be indeed commonplace in beef eaters) is quite low. Cardiovascular disease kills 1 million Americans annually.

The body can't consume milk, which explains exactly why around 70 percent of men are lactose-intolerant. If milk is removed from their diet, then they'll find their own skin-clearing upward (psoriasis, psoriasis (psoriasis), their allergies decreasing and their low levels of energy and low moods quitting - symptoms imputed to being flaxseed.

Professor t. Colin Campbell, who grew up on a dairy farm, also later became a professor of supplements. Campbell admits his research surprisingly resulted in evidence that diets high in animal-based protein resulted in the predominant levels of cancers and cardiovascular ailments in the current society. He hence admits he needed to reevaluate a few of the most precious beliefs (that eating beef, eggs and milk is great for the wellbeing) and clinics.

Many who follow the vegetarian diet that their own hair and claws have become fitter and stronger, their allergies have vanished, their acne and other skin issues have consumed, their energy have skyrocketed, extra weight dropped off plus so they finally have a new found zest for life. The high nutritional content of fruits and veggies, veggies, seeds, nuts, beans, beans, sea weed and wholegrains can be credited to those remarkable health benefits experienced in the dietplan. Additionally, dairy and meat products are no longer 'clogging up' their gastrointestinal tract.

Angela stokes was a obese young woman in her early twenties and had reached a huge 294lbs (133kg) at age 2-3. She had been still on the 'ordinary American diet' (i.e. She had been eating beef, legumes and eggs regularly) however she had been always feeling lethargic and sick. She had a diabetes frighten and endured thyroid issues. Stokes find out about the vegetarian food and shifted her diet plan to raw veganism overnight. She was a nutritious burden of 137lbs (62kg) for so many decades now and includes a deep zest forever.

Is your vegan diet healthy or un-healthy?

The discussion of perhaps the vegetarian diet is unhealthy or healthy isn't fresh. Nearly all folks will argue that someone who adopts veganism is going to undoubtedly be deficient in crucial nutrients found only in animal products and solutions, namely, animal-based protein. These individuals cherish the impression that milk will keep their bones strong and red meat will offer crucial protein to his or her muscles.

On another but there's really a tiny minority of folks (2 percent vegan and 5 percent vegetarian) who provide charge to the plant-based diet treating their acute health complications, permitting them to drop extra fat, unscrambling their allergies and skin, also giving them an remarkable zest for life.

Therefore according to both of these differences in remarks, just how can you determine if the vegetarian diet is healthy or unhealthy? All of it boils down, perhaps not things 'opinion,' but rather, on solid truth, signs, case studies and honest stories of real men and women.

Meat-eaters vs. Veggie eaters

Various studies imply that drinkers of reddish meat may die prematurely than people that eat little to no red meat. 1 us-based analysis of 120,000 people ascertained that drinkers of reddish meat are 20 percent more likely to die younger. Individuals that ate processed meats often encouraged this premature departure speed to a further 20% higher.

On another hand, michael f. Roizen, md, concludes that individuals that switch from eating beef products into vegetarian foods might easily add 13 years into their lifetime. Why? Vegetarians eat less animal fat and cholesterol, even whilst vegans have no animal fat or cholesterol. Professor t. Colin. Campbell (increased on a dairy farm) results from his experimental research program a beef and also dairy-free diet may both reverse and prevent 70 80 percent of disorder!

Weight reduction evidence

Fact: most dairy and meat products are high in calorie and fat content. By way of instance, 100g of steak comprises approximately 294 calories and 21g of fat (9% saturated) whilst 100g of cooked legumes comprises just 128 calories and 6.5gram of fat (0.8g saturated). Lamb contains 0g dietary fiber, even whilst 100g of lentils comprises 7.5grams fiber. Fiber enables one to feel fuller for more.

Evidence:

Angela stokes (aka'vegan raw food goddess') lost over 154lbs (70kg) in the vegan raw food diet. This remarkable woman, formerly morbidly obese, illustrates her fat reduction and new found zest for life into the vegetarian raw food and won't come back to the conventional American method of eating! Why? The benefits of the vegetarian diet (specially weight loss in angela's instance) are too great to offer up. Angel a embraced raw veganism immediately and never looked back as.

Physical benefits

Time and period again, men who embrace veganism proclaim their skin dries up (psoriasis, eczema, etc.)Their eyes become skinnier, their hair gets thicker and more fitter, their claws become stronger, their ability skyrocket and their allergies get rid of. Sound too good for decide to try, right?

These amazing health testimonials could result from the elevated nutrient and mineral material utilized in fruits and vegetables, seeds and nuts, legumes and beans, leafy greens and whole foods. The American dietetic association reasoned a vegetarian or vegetarian diet is definitely 'nutritionally sufficient,' and can offer numerous health advantages and cure or protect against certain diseases. Yes, even a 'well-orchestrated' vegetarian diet will offer you a generous number of crucial minerals and vitamins, therefore one's health is likely to improve.

What's your vegan diet unhealthy or healthy? You pick. People who have embraced veganism nevertheless, will always answer 'healthy' the benefits of the vegetarian diet obviously become apparent following one accomplishes this particular lifestyle.

The reality behind vegan fat reduction

There's an increasing amount of folks going to the diet for fat reduction purposes. Together with all these folks booming with this life, they have been setting a good example for many others and also inspiring them to additionally find this remarkable life style for themselves. It's undisputed that tens and thousands of men who've embraced veganism have undergone weight loss. Why is this true? Lets' look at 3 different variables below:

The calories are low

Processed food items, or foods that are fermented are low in calories and fat, where as beef in milk food are high in calorie and fat content. For that reason, with the comprehensive elimination of most meat and dairy food out of ones diet - weight loss ensues. It's inevitable that you may resolve.

1 research analyzed the calorie content of 5 plumped for non-vegan 5 and foods foods. Normally, the milk and meat foods comprised 315 calories per 100g, as the foods that were fermented comprised 170 calories per 100g.

This significant calorie gap can be credited to vegetarian foods normally becoming low in fat material. In the event that you should inspect the fat content of healthful foods, then you may also conclude that the vegetarian diet is certainly low-carb.

Non addictive

Studies suggest that fatty food items, foods that are fried and fatty foods possess a addictive character. This is the reason many men onto a normal diet over-eat till they feel so sick. They'll frequently have three portions of roast lamb, a massive milk shake, or another serving of this macaroni cheese. On the flip side, food onto the vegetarian diet includes a much more balanced taste and so, you won't be quite as ravenous once you're swallowing meals. With the removal of fatty acids and fatty dairy products and solutions, you could be certain your voracious, wild eating behaviours are going to undoubtedly be something of yesteryear! Yes, a lot of have managed to shed weight within the vegan diet due to the entire removal of addictive fatty and fatty animal-based food items!

The'i sense fitter' favorable effect

Each time someone adopts veganism, then they usually marvel at just how great they believe. Again and again, persons within the vegetarian diet having more energy, clearer skin, a much more joyful mood and a zest for life. This favorable effect of vegetarian foods frequently makes someone desire to keep with this diet program. They just don't want to return straight back to feeling awful back again! So, with the additional motivation to stay on the diet for a much longer time period, they have been allowing their own body to have healthy and to lose all surplus bodyfat. Really, weight loss in the vegan diet is inevitable!

21 Twenty One day meal-plan: plant-based

Day 1

Breakfast: apple cinnamon oatmeal (produce sufficient for wednesday)

Steak: cous-cous confetti salad (create enough to get one side with tomorrow's supper) and also carrot and red pepper soup (create sufficient for tomorrow's dinner)

Snack: toast with lemon cider vinegar and banana (easy option: banana or apple)

Dinner: hoppin' john salad along with kwick kale

Day 2

Protein: cereal, plant milk (your pick), and berries and banana

Lunch: vegan lemon beans (use wholegrain bread topped with lettuce, onion, tomato, along with your favourite chopped) and cup of carrot and red pepper soup (leftover from yesterday's lunch)

Snack: air-popped popcorn wrapped with curry powder or nutrient yeast

Dinner: southern beans and greens (throw on your left-over black-eyed legumes) with facet of cous-cous confetti salad (remaining yesterday's dinner)

Day 3

Breakfast: apple cinnamon oatmeal (leftover from monday; include chopped banana and think about having agave nectar, a tasty, low-glycemic indicator sweetener)

Steak: hummus and veggie sandwich (utilize pita or wholegrain bread, then spread with hummus, and high with lettuce, tomato, cucumbers, and also every other vegetables you need)

Snack: paper yogurt with berries dinner: curried lentil soup with left-over cous-cous confetti salad or a side salad (in the event you're making your side salad, contemplate greens, such as romaine or red leaf lettuce topped with celery, tomato, broccoli, onion, along with your treasured lowfat noodle dressing; yet an easy choice is cider vinegar, that is quite simple and also a little goes quite a very long way)

Day 4

Protein: cereal with plant milk (your pick) and frozen or fresh berries

Steak: vegan cup of soup (mcdougall's or amy's) using wholegrain bread

Snack: carrots and citrus dinner: kick-start diy (see kick-start diy hints at ending of menus): cous-cous, lentil, and kale

Day 5

Protein: smoothie day: fantastic fresh fruit smoothie

Steak: curried lentil soup or southern beans and greens

Snack: edamame or left-over hummus with carrots dinner: kick-start dining out: mexican

Day 6

Protein: blueberry buckwheat pancakes and facon bacon

Steak: easy-bean dip with ovenbaked tortilla chips and also a side dish (if you're making your side salad, then believe greens, such as romaine or red leaf lettuce topped with celery, tomato, broccoli, onion, along with your favourite low-carb noodle dressing; a simple choice is cider vinegar, that is quite simple and also a bit goes quite a very long way)

Dinner: easy stirfry using always great brown-rice (make additional for tomorrow's lunch rice batter; utilize frozen vegetables along with your leftover veggies from the week)

Dessert: chocolate raspberry mousse

Day 7

Protein: breakfast rice pudding (utilize leftover brown rice in the night's supper) or frozen waffles (using banana, berries, or equally)

Lunch: spinach salad with orange sesame dressing (include garbanzo beans) snack: ambrosia dinner: wholewheat pasta using simple marinara sauce (add broccoli, broccoli, broccoli, and also some other sour vegetables)

Day 8

Protein: cinnamon-raisin oatmeal

Lunch: missing egg sandwich (utilize whole grain bread and top with tomato and lettuce); include a side of ovenbaked tortilla chips and infant carrots

Snack: frozen mango chunks (obtain a bag of frozen cherry or eat fresh ones when available)

Dinner: barbeque-style portobellos over quinoa (quinoa is quick to create up and hamburgers in virtually no time) with fresh or steamed spinach

Day 9

Protein: cereal, plant milk, and also chopped strawberries on top

Steak: kick-start dining outside: salad pub gone crazy! Here's a tip for creating salad bar: pick a green salad, shirt using a bean, put in a grain along with a lot of vegetables, and then pick a low-carb vegan dressing table or keep it easy with balsamic vinegar (or even make your own salad in your home using romaine lettuce, garbanzo beans, tomato sauce, and balsamic vinegar)

Snack: oranges and raisins

Season: straightforward bean tacos with mexican corn salad (utilize leftover salad for tomorrow's dinner) dessert: berry mousse

Day 10

Protein: oatmeal with cherry and cinnamon (a dd plant milk)

Lunch: veggie burger with leftover mexican corn salad snack: carrot and citrus

Dinner: creamy broccoli soup with quinoa pilaf

Day 1-1

Protein: cereal with plant milk and a banana

Lunch: leftover missing egg sandwich and cup of leftover creamy broccoli soup

Snack: fresh grapes dinner: farm-house salad and left-over quinoa pilaf

Day-12

Morning meal: mango delight smoothie

Lunch: baked sweet potato together with left-over farm-house salad

Snack: air-popped pop corn using nutritional or curry yeast

Dinner: kick-start dining outside: japanese (attempt the carrot salad, edamame, a veggie sushi-roll, like a lemon roster or carrot rollup, along with miso soup)

Day 1 3

Morning meal: fruited breakfast quinoa and kick-start diy smoothie (utilize plant banana, milk, and some other fruit you've around; kick-start diy hints)

Lunch: immediately tomato salad and also asian guacamole using pita bread

Snack: edamame dinner: almost-instant black bean chili and easy corn bread muffins

Day 14

Protein: zucchini scramble and breakfast home fries

Lunch: taste salad (create left overs for tomorrow's dinner)

Snack: fresh fruit salad

Dinner: kick-start diy: beans, greens, legumes and grains (contemplate using broccoli, broccoli, and some other remaining kale or bok choy)

Day 1-5

Protein: oatmeal with berry (thaw frozen berry)

Lunch: leftover pasta salad using a piece of whole grain bread

Snack: orange pieces dinner: spicy thai soup (make extra if you'd like to work it in to lunch this week)

Day 16

Protein: frozen vegan waffles with berry and walnut syrup or cereal using plant fruit and milk

Steak: vegan cup of soup (or leftover spicy thai soup) with chopped sweet potato (try adding cinnamon ontop of one's candy potato)

Snack: red pepper hummus with uncooked veggies or pita bread

Dinner: buckwheat pasta with seitan and facet of sautéed kale dessert: chocolate banana smoothie

Day 17

Protein: oatmeal with banana or berries

Steak: kick-start dining out for lunch: oriental cuisine (search for your own broccoli and vegetable dishes with rice and also request them to be cooked or sauteed with light or no)

Snack: paper yogurt with fresh fruit dinner: lentil artichoke stew

Day 18

Protein: frozen vegan waffles using berry applesauce or cereal using plant fruit and milk

Lunch: leftover buckwheat pasta with seitan or even a veggie beans with wholewheat roll or bread, carrot, tomato, onions, and chopped

Snack: frozen grapes

Dinner: zippy yams along with bok choy using always great brown-rice

Day 1-9

Break fast: green goodie smoothie

Lunch: tomato, cucumber and basil salad with include can of garbanzo beans

Snack: berry applesauce (leftover from just eat an apple)

Dinner: kick-start dining out: italian

Day 20

Protein: spinach and mushroom frittata with facet of berry

Steak: quickie quesadillas snack: air-popped pop corn using curry powder or nutrient yeast

Dinner: chunky ratatouille sauce (conserve some sauce for lunch elsewhere) functioned over a grain, such as pasta, brown rice, couscous, quinoa, or orzo

Day 2-1

Protein: banana oat french toast with soysage (attempt gimme lean or a different dish manufacturer)

Lunch: homemade loaded baked potato with left-over chunky ratatouille sauce or create your own toppings, such as cauliflower, steamed broccoli, broccoli and legumes snack: cantaloupe or a different available fresh fruit

Dinner: hearty chili-mac with unsalted lettuce and mushrooms out of yesterday's spinach and mushroom frittata dessert: blueberry muffins (be sure to get for breakfast or just a bite weekly)

The transition to your vegan diet - slow and steady wins the race

Many people around the entire world are making serious changes in lifestyle so as to obtain their health in good state - and a lot of these individuals do so by way of the vegetarian dietplan. Yes, most folks are getting to be more and more conscious of the remarkable health benefits this diet offers, however, in many cases are frightened of creating the shift. Just how can they embrace veganism readily, without worrying? These hints are for people brand new to the vegan diet plan and also are needing to produce an effective transition into the vegan way of life.

The way to begin a vegan diet:

Measure 1 - do not worry!

Stressing in regards to the probable challenges and hardships of this vegan diet won't assist you in any manner, nor can it make you any closer to your objective. If you genuinely want to embrace the veganism life style, (even when you're fearful only a little) - don't stress! This is definitely an important suggestion for your newcomer vegans, because so most appear to worry too much and pass up of a great deal of joy this amazing travel has to offer you!

Measure two - you really do not have to really go vegan immediately.

Some individuals are able to ditch their previous way of life and embrace a new one immediately. I commend persons similar to this, for that is something which a number people would love to complete - but only might not. For nearly all people, embracing a brand new life style does take patience, time, and also making small steps towards their own objective. Don't despair if that really is you!

Building a slow hurry into the vegan diet plan is advised.

Whilst the famous saying goes 'slow and steady wins the race' therefore making slow but steady modifications to your daily diet helps slowly ingrain your fresh life style in your brain, and you'll do it at an appropriate, flat-rate rate! Giving time to become accustomed to the tiny measures and eliminations of this vegan diet is essential for the novice vegetarian!

The practice of removal

The subsequent 7 foods needs to be eradicated, individually, at an appropriate pace: 1). Red-meat. 2. White meat (poultry) 3. Fish & fish. 4. Cheese. 5. Eggs. 6. Butter/cream. 7. Milk

Should you gradually eliminate those foods your transition into the vegan diet will probably soon be more gratifying and stress-free! Since you accomplish each stage of removal, you should attempt to locate some yummy recipes that adapt for the brand new dietary wants. It's possible to discover a number of vegan/vegan transition recipes online, either out of blogs, websites, or professional vegetarian recipe e books. For all those new to this veganism life style, finding yummy and easy-to-make recipes is vital to help you stay motivated and appreciating with your meal!

CHAPTER 7

STRATEGIES FOR YOUR BEGINNER VEGAN - GUIDELINES ON HOW TO BEGIN A VEGAN DIET

Earning the transition into a vegetarian diet for the very first time might be equally daunting yet exciting at precisely the exact same moment. The newcomer vegetarian frequently has lots of questions or doubts concerning it life style they are working to get replies for. Below is an inventory of 10 tips for people that are new to the vegetarian dietplan, emphasizing the best way best to smoothly begin a vegetarian diet plan and also the way to be certain the transition into becoming vegetarian is just as easy as achievable.

Inch. Research & gather information

Before you create any sort of life style modification, it's always a fantastic strategy to do plenty of research ahead. In that way, you're going to learn precisely what to anticipate. You want to assemble info on which vegans do and also do not eat, what benefits you're to moving vegan, what barriers and struggles vegans face, etc.,. You may thank yourself in the future for the detailed investigation.

2. What would you like to attain?

For your newcomer vegan, I advise them to jot down in writing just what they would like to reach the vegan way of life. May it be weight loss, to clean skin conditions (e.g.: psoriasis, eczema, psoriasis) to attain inner peace, to lessen allergies, even to reverse chronic disease, to concentrate better, to save the planet, animal rights, etc., - no matter your reasons are to producing the transition into the vegetarian diet, and write them down to paper. Stick them at which you're able to observe them every single day like on the ice box.

3. Find superior recipes

It's totally necessary to discover and collect some fantastic vegetarian meals, as you're going to do plenty of distinct cooking from today on. You want to obtain some easy and quick recipes to the changing times when you're just too tired or busy to cook whatever elaborate. Additionally gather an extensive range of vegetarian recipes such as rice breakfast meals, lunches, dinners and snacks, cakes, pieces, desserts, etc... Find your recipes on line, buy a vegetarian recipe e book - you pick, just be certain that you have your own vegan recipe well-prepared for if you're beginning your own fresh vegan way of life.

4. Let family & friends know

Let your cherished ones understand whenever you make your choice to become vegetarian. This will guarantee that after you see them or any time they see you personally, food won't be a challenge given that they've been already advised about your brand new dietplan.

5. Be prepared for cravings

If you cease eating food items, you are going to necessarily have cravings for food every so often. Be ready for this and be certain that to have any nutritious snacks or frozen baking readily accessible and that means you never cave. Locate some recipes too for "vegan clones " your favorite snacks and meals (notice: professional vegan chefs've written an range of recipe e books to accommodate for the cravings).

6. Know your own vegan food brands

Now the supermarkets and health shops tailor to the wants of this dish, and that means you shouldn't have any trouble finding meat-free, dairy-free foods and snacks like vegan cheese, broccoli, vegan chocolate, health pubs, "bacon " and cereal. Try them out and also have acquainted with your favorites.

7. Stay motivated on the web

You will find lots of vegan online service groups, chat rooms and blogs which you may go to and socialize with fellow vegans on the web. This can allow one stay motivated, motivated, and may even allow one to see that you're perhaps not the sole dish around earth!

8. Love your own fresh fruit & vegetable shopping

You may end up eating far more fresh produce today that you're vegetarian. Locate some vegetable and fruit supermarket or food stores which deliver quality produce in a sensible price. Remember that supermarkets are frequently pricier. Enjoy choosing your fresh produce and produce your vegetable and vegetable buying a more calming experience!

9. Bake your very own healthy treats & snacks

As you will be restricted by purchasing snacks and candies out at restaurants and cafes, bake your vegan treats such as brownies, cakes, pieces and sandwiches. Bake a whole batch weekly and then freeze individual portions for if you want a treat. Once more, it is possible to get a large amount of vegetarian recipes on the web by blogs, websites, or recipe e books.

10. Do not quit easily

The transition into the vegan life is the toughest at the start. After a time, it is going to get easier and easier until it will become second nature for you. Therefore for the newcomer vegan or people relatively new to the vegan way of life, my advice isn't to offer up right off but to present your new life style a reasonable chance. It's probable that after a couple of weeks you'll be exceedingly thankful that you never threw in the towel! The advantages and advantages of the life style consistently outweigh any challenges you can face from time to time!

For all those who need to produce the transition into a vegetarian diet there are 3 steps outlined below that you need to attempt to follow along with for your novice vegan, the notion of moving vegan overnight may seem very frightening. Be confident nevertheless. That you don't need to create this life style change immediately, however you may make the transition slowly. The next 3 measures demonstrate how to begin a vegetarian diet and gradually.

Get informed

Before beginning any life style modification, it's very important that you obtain your self-well-informed. This implies exploring everything you could imagine in regards to the vegetarian dietplan. Thorough research is vital for the newcomer vegan since this may notify you exactly what to expect, which challenges might emerge, the way to take care of the social struggles to be vegetarian, the way to remain motivated, exactly what health benefits you may anticipate, what spiritual and psychological influences could occur, etc.,.

Get motivated

For all those not used to the vegetarian diet (vegan starters!) Or into the notion of it you have to grab your self-motivated! I am talking about, you have to really end up straightened and excited about moving vegan. Why? Becoming excited and excited to begin your brand new vegan travel may help ensure victory and certainly will allow you to strong when struggles and barriers arise on the way.

Therefore just how do you get yourself inspired?

Read achievement stories of other people. Look for success stories out of other folk who've uttered similar advantages from the vegetarian diet (to all those advantages of that you may love to have). You may find loads of excellent success stories on you tube, which can be truly inspirational!

How else could you get inspired?

Many people think that meals onto the vegetarian diet is more really boring. Well they have been mistaken! You're able to end up motivated to start the vegan transition from collecting and finding a range of tasty, mouthwatering vegan recipes. You ought to amass a number of vegetarian recipes such as recipes for vegetarian foods, lunches, breakfasts, snacks, cakes, quick & easy vegetarian foods, desserts, etc.. Collect your recipes on line, either from blogs, sites, or even professional vegan recipe e books.

Begin your transition

Gradually start the transition into the diet. One at a time, and rather from the next sequence, remove these foods out of the daily diet

Inch. Red-meat

2. White beef (poultry)

3. Fish and fish

4. Cheese

5. Eggs

6. Butter/cream

7. Milk

Do not attempt to rush into the following stage of this transition in the event that you aren't ready. By way of instance, if you're around point 3 of fish and fish, however you're finding this point hard, don't panic! Move ahead into the following removal platform at a comfy pace whenever you're prepared. Bear in mind, slow and steady wins the race!

A vegan diet program plan is worth another look

Did you realize that the typical man will spend 5 decades of their own lives only eating? Since i'm now in my 60 th year it'd be safe to stateIqualify as a expert on ingestion. It takes 4 years to find a level and you do not devote every waking hour. Surely right now i've earned my schooling in confront id.

Lately my spouse and I left the transition into a vegetarian eating plan. She is exactly about any of it. I sometimes will throw a turkey hamburger however typically we're toeing the vegetarian lineup.

A few days past as both folks were talking our daily diet conditions that I inquired that a very dumb question. What is the distinction between vegetarians and vegans? Are they in the exact same or is there any gaps in how that they approach vegetables?

With no hesitation my spouse retorted that vegans do not consume milk product. Imagine my terror once I thought that ice-cream was an endangered species within my own daily diet.

Within moments I thrilled Google and started an internet hunt to suppress my fascination about veganism. Is that a whole lot of weirdos...holdovers from the hippie motion? Are you currently members of peta? Or...are they on something I have only missed out in my own years of gorging myself?

After all, because we've embraced a much healthier lifestyle it seemed only reasonable that I find more information about the dietplan. So what can a vegetarian eat? Can a vegetarian diet program take our very best interest?

A standard vegan diet includes seeds, legumes, soy products, nuts, produce. Okay. I am with you thus far. That is what we eat.

An average daily routine comprises fresh fruit. The mid-day and evening meals contain fresh vegetables and salads as well as steamed or sautéed veggies and grains.

The vegan diet plan spicy foods which are full of fatty foods, animal protein and cholesterol nonetheless includes foods high in potassium, fiber, carbohydrates, magnesium, and calcium.

So that is an breakdown of the things they do eat and the things they don't really eat. However, which will be the advantages? Check out this. A vegetarian diet will help to lessen the probability of severe health issues such as those diseases most of us would like to prevent...cancer, cardiovascular disease, diabetes, obesity, arthritis, obesity, diabetes, kidney issues, higher blood pressure, and also aging.

There's nevertheless a word of warning which is included with the diet. What you stop trying...meat, eggs, milk, etc.. Eliminates significant nourishment from the daily diet. Ergo, if you aren't attentive to acquire a excellent understanding of the way the vegetarian diet operates you might do any severe damage to the physique. It isn't the type of diet which you jump right into and also learn in the future. You could possibly even have to count calories for some time simply to ensure you are receiving enough fuel to the human own body.

Vegan proponents suggest doing your own homework. Learn the fundamentals connected to the diet before investing it. Subsequently ease into it slowly in the place of simply quitting your previous diet "cold turkey "pardon the pun.

Fish and fish provide our own bodies with necessary nourishment and omega 3 fatty acids that are essential. Finding replacements for all these nutritional supplements pose challenging. So it's crucial to master all of the vegetarian replacements for your nourishment obtained from beef as well as other non-vegan food solutions. The most usual replacement foods such as meat include tofu, sietan and tempeh.

You likely understand about kale but could be new to sietan and tempeh. Tempeh is a fermented product (produced from legumes or soybeans) originally from Indonesia with a slightly sweet feel and a solid flavor. Sietan is wheat germ free and can also be referred to as the titles wheat-meat, mock duck, also gluten free meat.

Additionally, there are varying strategies into this diet program. By way of instance, you will find a few people who eat around 75 percent in the food raw. Undoubtedly that could be a significant challenge for almost all of people however it's infact that the most economical manner we can eat.

For a lot of us veganism can be a fresh thing but it's been around for quite a very long moment. The vegetarian diet program is hauled in early hinduism and it has turned into a frequent fixture at the indian life style as prior to the christian age. Really, for a few, the dietary plan is regarded as perfect for spiritual advancement.

We've got a inclination to deny that which we do not know and i'd suppose that lots of men and women refuse any diet which eliminates good old fashioned meat and potatoes. But we would be wise to supply the vegetarian diet a closer glance.

CONCLUSION

Just because there's evidence the keto diet regime works and produces fast, evidence against it (specially longterm) is just starting to accumulate also.

For you personally, its own benefits reduction overtime, and you also lose not just surplus fat however slim down too. Secondly, it almost undoubtedly increases your chance of developing nonalcoholic fatty liver disorder, which may cause cirrhosis. Last, and above all, studies have revealed it might increase cardiovascular disease, that may, in turn, increase your chance of developing cardiovascular diseases, plus in addition, it increases the danger of respiratory and colon cancer.

Thanks to them potential health hazards, it's not a good idea to call home with this particular diet longterm.

The keto diet and seniors

Aging ought to no way stop some one from moving to a keto diet in reality, it might be better for elderly adults. In any case, way too many carbohydrates and an excessive amount of processed foods never assist improve older nutrition.

You will find lots of advantages of seniors who opt to try out a keto diet to drop weight. The principal benefits are connected to encouraging physical and mental health at any given age.

Here are a few of the most notable benefits of keeping up a ketogenic diet

Defeating insulin resistance -- lots of older persons are too heavy and coping with insulin-related conditions such as diabetes.

Increased bone health -- osteoporosis symptoms might also be relieved by means of a keto diet in 2 manners: by lowering the creation of radicals, that restrict absorption, and swallowing a broad assortment of foods that the full of micro nutrients, in the place of being over loaded to a certain micro nutrient (calcium).

Slimming illness -- this can help to improve the symptoms due to joint problems such as arthritis and other inflammatory problems.

Avoiding nutrient deficiencies -- shared ketogenic diet programs are full of iron, vitamin b 12, fat-soluble vitamins such as vitamin d, vitamin and animal proteins. The exclusion this may be your vegan keto diet, even where in fact the deficient vitamins and nutrients should be offered from plant sources.

Pairing blood glucose this is essential not just for diabetes also for brain-related conditions for example Alzheimer's disease, dementia, diabetes, and Parkinson's disease.

Ketosis could probably repair a number of this damage brought on by treating our own bodies seriously. But when it comes to older adults, this may impact their wellbeing, as well. The ketogenic diet might help seniors improve their wellbeing to ensure they could thrive, get sick more frequently, and feel pain in their subsequent years.